Unraveling Parsonage-Turner: Comprehensive Insights on Symptoms and Treatment

Dustin Gross

Published by Dustin Gross, 2025.

UNRAVELING PARSONAGE-TURNER: COMPREHENSIVE INSIGHTS ON SYMPTOMS AND TREATMENT

First edition. August 26, 2025.

ISBN: 979-8230117162

Written by Dustin Gross.

Table of Contents

Glossary of Terms

One of the most frustrating parts of encountering a medical diagnosis is the flood of acronyms and jargon that come with it. This glossary is designed to demystify the most common terms you will see throughout the guide. The goal is not to turn you into a neurologist overnight, but to give you the confidence to follow discussions, ask smart questions, and understand your care plan.

- **PTS (Parsonage-Turner Syndrome):** A disorder of the peripheral nerves, especially the brachial plexus, usually triggered by immune or inflammatory events. Also called *neuralgic amyotrophy*.
- **Brachial Plexus:** A network of nerves that originates from the spinal cord in the neck (C5–T1 roots) and controls movement and sensation in the shoulder, arm, and hand.
- **Plexopathy:** Damage or dysfunction of a plexus (a bundle of nerves).
- **Atrophy:** Wasting or shrinking of muscle due to loss of nerve supply.
- **Winged Scapula:** A shoulder blade that protrudes out like a wing due to paralysis of stabilizing muscles, most often the serratus anterior (innervated by the long thoracic nerve).
- **EMG (Electromyography):** A test that measures the electrical activity of muscles to assess whether nerves are functioning normally.
- **NCS (Nerve Conduction Study):** A test that stimulates nerves with small electrical impulses to measure how quickly and effectively signals travel. Often paired with EMG.
- **MRN (Magnetic Resonance Neurography):** A specialized MRI technique that visualizes nerves themselves, not just bones and muscles. Useful for identifying constrictions or torsions in PTS.
- **AIN (Anterior Interosseous Nerve):** A branch of the median nerve in the forearm; injury causes inability to pinch thumb and index finger.

- **PIN (Posterior Interosseous Nerve):** A branch of the radial nerve; injury causes finger drop without sensory loss.
- **ROM (Range of Motion):** The extent to which a joint can move in all directions.
- **Neuropathic Pain:** Pain arising from nerves themselves rather than tissue injury. Described as burning, stabbing, or electric.
- **Corticosteroids (Prednisone):** Anti-inflammatory medication sometimes used early in PTS to dampen immune attack. Evidence is mixed.
- **Neurolysis:** Surgical freeing of a nerve from constricting tissue.
- **Nerve Transfer:** A surgical technique in which a healthy donor nerve is rerouted to restore function to a paralyzed muscle.
- **QuickDASH:** A validated questionnaire measuring disability of the arm, shoulder, and hand, often used to track functional recovery.

Disclaimer

This book is intended as an informational guide, not as a medical prescription. The condition known as Parsonage-Turner Syndrome is complex, variable, and often unpredictable. While we draw upon the most current scientific evidence and expert consensus available as of 2025, the field continues to evolve, and every patient's journey is unique.

Reading this book does not create a doctor–patient relationship. It is not meant to replace individualized evaluation, diagnosis, or treatment by a licensed healthcare professional. Decisions about your health, including medications, physical therapy, imaging, or surgery, must be made in consultation with clinicians who know your history and can examine you directly.

We also acknowledge the limits of research in this field. Unlike conditions such as diabetes or hypertension, there are no large randomized controlled trials guiding most aspects of PTS care. Treatments such as early corticosteroids, IVIG, or surgery for hourglass constrictions are supported by observational studies, case series, and expert opinion rather than definitive proof. That means recommendations often reflect probabilities, not guarantees.

The authors, contributors, and publisher disclaim liability for any adverse outcomes arising from the application of information contained in this book. Use it as a companion, a translator, and a source of questions—but not as your sole compass.

If you are reading this while in acute pain, struggling to lift your arm, or worried about your breathing, please seek immediate medical attention. There are urgent red flags that require prompt evaluation: difficulty breathing, bilateral weakness, rapidly progressing paralysis, or new neurologic deficits. Do not wait to see how things evolve.

This book exists to empower you with knowledge and perspective. Take it into your appointments, share sections with your therapists or family, and highlight the questions that matter most to you. Information is power, but only when paired with partnership and care.

Introduction

If you are holding this book, chances are you—or someone you love—has been swept into the whirlwind of Parsonage-Turner Syndrome. Maybe you woke up one night with pain so searing it felt like fire under your skin, and you were told by urgent care that it was "probably a muscle strain." Maybe weeks later your shoulder muscles began melting away, and you could no longer lift a coffee cup or comb your hair. Maybe you were sent from orthopedic surgeon to physical therapist to rheumatologist before anyone even whispered the words "neuralgic amyotrophy."

This journey is frightening, frustrating, and often isolating. But you are not alone, and you are not imagining it. PTS is real. It is under-recognized, but it is real. And this book is designed to help you navigate it.

The chapters that follow will walk you through the basics of the condition, the science behind it, the tests you may undergo, the treatments available, and—most importantly—what life with PTS actually looks like. Along the way, you will hear from composite patient stories that reflect the lived experiences of many people with this condition. You will find sidebars, call-out boxes, and checklists designed to help you prepare for appointments, ask better questions, and track your progress.

We will not sugarcoat the challenges. Recovery is often slow, uneven, and incomplete. Some patients regain most of their function within a year; others are left with residual deficits that require adaptation. Pain may fade, but fatigue, weakness, and asymmetry can persist. These realities deserve honesty, because unrealistic expectations breed disappointment.

At the same time, we will not abandon hope. Many patients find creative ways to adapt, to regain independence, and even to thrive. Physical therapy, occupational strategies, pacing, and community support can transform despair into resilience. Small wins—buttoning a shirt, throwing a ball, sleeping through the night without stabbing pain—become milestones worth celebrating.

Think of this book as a companion on your journey. It cannot take the pain away, but it can keep you from walking blindfolded. It can connect you to the larger story of PTS, where science is advancing, awareness is spreading, and patients are finding each other. It can help you reclaim a sense of agency in a condition that too often strips it away.

So, begin here. Read at your own pace. Mark the sections that resonate. Share the glossary with your family so they can follow the conversation. Bring the appendices to your appointments. Let the knowledge empower you, not overwhelm you.

Your journey with Parsonage-Turner Syndrome is uniquely yours. But you do not have to make it in silence, and you do not have to make it without tools. This book is one such tool.

Chapter 1: Understanding Parsonage-Turner Syndrome

Parsonage-Turner Syndrome. At first encounter, the name might sound like the surname of two stern professors you would avoid at a university faculty party, but in reality it represents one of the most painful, disorienting, and under-recognized neurological conditions encountered in medicine. Also known as neuralgic amyotrophy, PTS is not a quaint textbook curiosity but an immune-triggered disorder of the peripheral nerves, most often involving the brachial plexus. For a long time it has worn the false label of "rare," lurking in obscure case reports and specialty clinics. Yet the closer the medical world looks, the more evident it becomes: this condition is far from vanishingly rare. It is simply hidden in plain sight, misdiagnosed, dismissed, or ignored until it wreaks havoc on lives. Understanding it begins with stripping away myths and carefully laying out what it is, how it manifests, and why early recognition can profoundly shape outcomes.

Defining the Syndrome

Parsonage-Turner Syndrome is an acute neuropathy, meaning a sudden attack on the nerves outside the brain and spinal cord. Unlike chronic neuropathies such as diabetic peripheral neuropathy, which develop gradually, PTS is abrupt and dramatic. Patients are often blindsided. One day they may feel perfectly normal, and the next they are slammed by pain that seems wildly disproportionate to any activity they performed. No awkward lift, no sporting accident, no fall. Just a lightning strike of pain that comes on without reason. This is the hallmark: abrupt severe pain in the shoulder, upper arm, or sometimes neck, which then evolves into weakness and wasting of muscles supplied by the affected nerves.

The trajectory is so consistent across patients that clinicians often speak of it as a three-act play. First act: searing pain. Second act: focal weakness and atrophy. Third act: long recovery, sometimes redemptive, sometimes incomplete. The plot may differ in detail, but the structure is recognizable. For this reason, many physicians who have seen it once never forget it—yet too many never see it, because the diagnosis is never considered.

The nerve injury in PTS arises from an immune-mediated process. In idiopathic cases, the body's own immune system turns on the peripheral nerves, attacking them after being triggered by a viral infection, vaccination, childbirth, or even surgical stress. In hereditary cases, a genetic predisposition makes nerves more vulnerable, particularly due to mutations in the SEPT9 gene. The result is inflammation, demyelination (loss of protective nerve insulation), and axonal injury (damage to the conducting core of the nerve). When a nerve loses its function, the muscles it controls weaken and waste away.

Understanding this process gives patients one critical truth: the weakness that follows the pain is not laziness, deconditioning, or simply "babying the arm." It is a direct consequence of nerve injury. Muscles cannot obey commands if their wiring is cut, no matter how much willpower or effort is applied.

The Classic Progression

The first phase, acute pain, is legendary for its ferocity. Patients often describe it in metaphors: "like being stabbed with an ice pick," "like fire burning inside the joint," "like lightning bolts every time I moved." It is sharp, stabbing, electric, relentless, and typically worse at night. Over-the-counter pain relievers rarely bring relief. Narcotics may dull it temporarily, but the pain often breaks through. This phase can last days to weeks, and as it begins to subside, the second phase begins, leaving devastation in its wake.

Weakness appears, sometimes insidiously, sometimes overnight. A person discovers that they cannot lift their arm overhead, cannot grip a fork tightly, cannot snap their fingers. The pattern of weakness depends on which nerves are affected. The long thoracic nerve produces winging of the scapula, the shoulder blade jutting outward from the ribcage. The suprascapular nerve causes weakness of the rotator cuff, limiting shoulder rotation. The anterior interosseous nerve makes it impossible to pinch thumb to index finger, leaving fine motor tasks impossible. The posterior interosseous nerve results in finger drop, making typing or playing instruments futile. These are not theoretical; they are daily functional losses that alter the fabric of life.

Over weeks, visible atrophy sets in. Muscles shrink, divots form under the skin where mass used to be, and asymmetry becomes striking. For patients, this visible wasting compounds the emotional toll, as it provides a daily mirror of the damage. This phase can last months, during which function is impaired and adaptations must be made.

Finally comes recovery, the most variable phase of all. Nerves regenerate slowly, and while some people experience remarkable improvement within a year, others remain disabled for much longer. Recovery may be partial; residual weakness, fatigue, and altered mechanics are common. In idiopathic PTS, about three-quarters of patients recover significant function, but many are left with subtle deficits. In hereditary PTS, recurrences are common and cumulative damage accumulates. Rehabilitation, physical therapy, and sometimes surgery play roles in shaping this long road.

Epidemiology: Not as Rare as You Think

For decades, PTS was taught as a rare zebra diagnosis. Medical students memorized it for exams but rarely expected to encounter it in practice. Older textbooks cite an incidence of two per 100,000 per year, a number repeated without question. Yet prospective studies in the last decade have shattered that myth. When researchers systematically evaluated patients presenting with acute shoulder pain in primary care, they discovered that up to one in every thousand developed PTS. This means that thousands of cases are occurring each year, but most are written off as "rotator cuff tear," "cervical radiculopathy," or simply "muscle strain."

The consequence is profound under-diagnosis. Patients bounce between orthopedic surgeons, physical therapists, rheumatologists, and pain specialists, often for months, before someone recognizes the pattern. By then, valuable time is lost, and opportunities for early intervention have slipped away.

Epidemiology also reveals certain demographics. Men are affected slightly more than women. Age of onset ranges from adolescence to old age, but most cases cluster between ages 20 and 60. No occupational group is immune; both athletes and office workers, manual laborers and musicians, have been struck. Hereditary cases often cluster in families, sometimes masquerading as "bad shoulders" or "family weakness" until genetic testing reveals the underlying SEPT9 mutation.

The "rare" label has done more harm than good. It discourages awareness, reduces funding, and isolates patients. The reality is that PTS is common enough that every primary care physician, orthopedic surgeon, and neurologist should be able to recognize it. The challenge is not rarity, but recognition.

Who Gets It and Why

One of the most unsettling aspects of PTS is its unpredictability. A healthy person with no prior medical issues can be struck overnight. Others have identifiable triggers. Infections—particularly viral illnesses—are among the most common. Vaccinations, including flu and COVID-19 vaccines, have been implicated in some cases, though the benefit of vaccination far outweighs the small risk of triggering an immune reaction. Surgical procedures, childbirth, and intense physical stress have also been reported as triggers.

The underlying mechanism is believed to be immune dysregulation: the body mounts a defense against a perceived invader, but mistakenly targets nerve tissue. The brachial plexus, with its long, branching pathways and delicate fascicular structure, seems particularly vulnerable. In hereditary cases, SEPT9 mutations weaken the scaffolding of nerves, making them more prone to injury.

Interestingly, PTS is not confined to the brachial plexus. Though most cases involve the shoulder and arm, some involve the lumbosacral plexus, leading to leg weakness, or cranial nerves, leading to facial or vocal cord involvement. The syndrome is a reminder that the nervous system is interconnected, and immune attacks do not always follow neat boundaries.

A Brief History

The syndrome takes its name from Maurice Parsonage and John Turner, British physicians who in 1948 published a landmark series describing 136 cases of acute brachial neuritis with pain, weakness, and wasting. Their meticulous clinical observations cemented the condition in medical literature. Yet even before them, nineteenth-century physicians described similar phenomena, though lacking the tools to localize the problem to the plexus.

For decades after 1948, the syndrome remained a quiet corner of neurology, overshadowed by more common disorders like multiple sclerosis or Guillain-Barré syndrome. It was considered an oddity, something that might appear once in a career. But the last twenty years have revolutionized understanding. Advances in imaging—especially magnetic resonance neurography and high-resolution ultrasound—revealed that in many cases, the culprit is not diffuse inflammation alone but focal constrictions. These "hourglass constrictions" are sites where the nerve twists and narrows, choking off function. This discovery redefined the syndrome and created new possibilities: surgical intervention to release the constriction or transfer nerves before irreversible damage occurs.

This history illustrates a broader lesson in medicine: diseases once dismissed as curiosities can, with better tools, be revealed as common, important, and treatable. PTS is a perfect example.

Figures in Words: The Brachial Plexus Map

Imagine the spinal cord as a tree trunk and the nerves as branches extending out to control the arms. From the spinal cord in the neck emerge five roots—C5, C6, C7, C8, and T1. These roots braid together into trunks, then divide into divisions, regroup as cords, and finally branch into peripheral nerves. This intricate weaving is the brachial plexus. It is the wiring harness of the upper limb, and like any complex wiring system, it is vulnerable to faults at multiple points.

The long thoracic nerve runs along the chest wall, innervating the serratus anterior muscle that holds the scapula against the ribcage. Injury here produces the striking winged scapula. The suprascapular nerve powers the supraspinatus and infraspinatus muscles, critical for shoulder abduction and rotation. The anterior interosseous nerve, a branch of the median, controls fine pinch. The posterior interosseous nerve, a branch of the radial, extends the fingers. Each of these is a thread in the plexus tapestry, and in PTS, any of them can be selectively attacked. This patchiness is what makes the syndrome so variable and so confusing to those unfamiliar with it.

Why Early Recognition Matters

The difference between early recognition and delayed diagnosis is the difference between opportunity and regret. In the acute phase, corticosteroids may shorten the course of pain and possibly improve recovery, though data are mixed. More importantly, identifying the condition early prevents unnecessary surgeries. Too many patients undergo rotator cuff repairs or cervical spine surgeries that do nothing for their real problem. Early recognition channels them toward appropriate care: pain control, electrodiagnostic testing at the right time, imaging if needed, and rehabilitation strategies to protect joints and prevent maladaptive mechanics.

For those with constrictions, early detection opens the door to surgical intervention before muscles are irreversibly lost. For those without surgical lesions, early referral to rehabilitation helps maintain mobility and function. And for all, early recognition validates the suffering and provides a name. A diagnosis, even when it comes with uncertainty, is powerful. It ends the gaslighting of "it's just stress" and replaces it with legitimacy.

This is why awareness matters—not just among neurologists, but among family physicians, orthopedists, therapists, and patients themselves. The earlier PTS is recognized, the better the chance of optimizing recovery.

Conclusion

Parsonage-Turner Syndrome is more than a neurological curiosity. It is a common, under-recognized, and often disabling condition that deserves serious attention. Defined by a triad of abrupt pain, focal weakness, and gradual recovery, it reshapes lives. Its incidence is higher than previously believed, its triggers diverse, and its outcomes variable. History has brought it from obscurity to recognition, and modern imaging has opened new frontiers in treatment.

To understand PTS is to recognize it quickly, treat it realistically, and support those who endure it. In the chapters that follow, we will dive into the details: how to identify its symptoms, how to pursue the right diagnostic workup, what the latest research reveals, what treatments exist, and how to live with and beyond the condition. The journey ahead is complex, but knowledge is the first compass. This chapter has laid the foundation. The next will build upon it by teaching you how to identify symptoms—those first clues that distinguish Parsonage-Turner Syndrome from the many mimics that so often steal the spotlight.

Chapter 2: Identifying Symptoms

If Chapter 1 was about naming the storm, Chapter 2 is about reading the clouds before the downpour floods your life. Parsonage-Turner Syndrome announces itself in dramatic fashion, but because its signs overlap with more common shoulder and neck problems, patients are often misdiagnosed at the very moment when recognition matters most. The key to navigating this condition is learning to distinguish its specific pattern of pain, weakness, and variability. These clues are not subtle when you know what to look for, but they can be easily lost in the shuffle of a busy clinic or buried under the weight of misleading imaging reports. To identify PTS is to spot the difference between a twisted ankle and a fractured bone—both painful, both disabling, but very different in what they mean for the future.

The Pain That Starts It All

Pain is the first and loudest symptom of PTS. It is not just uncomfortable—it is overwhelming. Patients often use words like stabbing, burning, or tearing to describe it. Some say it feels as if a knife is lodged in the shoulder blade, twisting with every breath. Others compare it to an electrical storm firing inside their muscles. Unlike musculoskeletal pain, which can often be eased with rest or repositioning, PTS pain is relentless. It tends to worsen at night, robbing patients of sleep and leaving them physically and emotionally exhausted. The cruel irony is that this initial pain often misleads both patient and physician. Because it centers around the shoulder, it is mistaken for a rotator cuff tear, frozen shoulder, or bursitis. Anti-inflammatory medications and rest provide little relief, leaving people confused as to why their "injury" feels so disproportionate.

The duration of the pain phase varies. For some, it is an intense but short-lived storm, lasting a week or two before subsiding. For others, it stretches on for several weeks, gnawing at the edges of daily function. Yet what unites almost all patients is that once the pain begins to fade, a new and equally devastating problem emerges: weakness. This transition is the pivot point of PTS, the moment when the condition reveals itself for what it really is—not a joint problem, but a nerve problem.

Weakness and Its Delayed Arrival

Unlike traumatic injuries where weakness and pain arrive simultaneously, PTS weakness is delayed. Often, patients recall that only after the worst of the pain receded did they notice that certain movements had disappeared from their repertoire. They tried to lift their arm overhead and failed. They tried to pinch their thumb and index finger together and found the fingers simply would not obey. They noticed that a once-firm handshake had gone limp, or that typing felt like an impossible marathon of fatigue. This delayed onset is one of the hallmark features of PTS.

The weakness is nerve-specific, not general. Which muscles fail depends on which nerves have been attacked. If the long thoracic nerve is injured, the patient develops a winged scapula—the shoulder blade jutting backward like a loose hinge on a door. If the anterior interosseous nerve is involved, fine motor tasks collapse, making it impossible to hold a pen correctly or form the "OK" sign with thumb and finger. The suprascapular nerve robs the shoulder of rotation and abduction, making daily tasks like combing hair or reaching into cupboards impossible. The posterior interosseous nerve leaves fingers limp, unable to extend. The variety of presentations confuses clinicians, but for those who know the syndrome, the patchiness of weakness is one of its defining features.

What makes this phase even more demoralizing is the visible muscle wasting that follows. Within weeks, muscle mass shrinks, revealing bony contours and hollowed spaces where strength used to reside. Patients often find this deeply unsettling. The atrophy is not just cosmetic—it signals that the nerve is no longer feeding the muscle, and unless regeneration occurs, the loss may be permanent. This stark visibility is part of what makes PTS such a traumatic diagnosis.

The Strange Variability of Nerve Involvement

PTS is nothing if not unpredictable. It is not confined to one neat anatomical box, and its variability often fools both patients and doctors. Some people experience isolated palsy of a single nerve, leaving them with a narrowly defined deficit. Others find multiple nerves affected in a patchwork pattern. Still others experience involvement outside the brachial plexus entirely, such as the phrenic nerve, which controls the diaphragm, or the recurrent laryngeal nerve, which supplies the vocal cords. These less common but dramatic variants produce symptoms like unexplained breathlessness, sleep apnea, or sudden hoarseness. For a patient already reeling from shoulder pain, discovering that they cannot breathe deeply or that their voice has changed adds another layer of fear.

This variability is both a curse and a clue. It is a curse because it makes diagnosis harder—few clinicians think "nerve disorder" when faced with hoarseness after a cold. But it is a clue because very few other conditions produce such a bizarre and selective patchwork of deficits. Recognizing this patchiness helps distinguish PTS from mimics like cervical radiculopathy, which usually follows a predictable root distribution, or rotator cuff tears, which affect mechanical strength without nerve-specific wasting.

When to Seek Help

In any neurological disorder, there are moments when waiting is acceptable and moments when immediate medical attention is essential. PTS has its share of red flags. Patients should seek urgent evaluation if they develop difficulty breathing, especially if they notice shortness of breath lying flat or sudden worsening of sleep apnea symptoms. Bilateral cases—where both sides of the body are involved—are also concerning and warrant immediate specialist referral. Rapidly progressing weakness, where multiple muscles fail over days, should trigger urgent investigation to rule out more widespread conditions. Severe scapular winging that prevents normal function should not be dismissed as "posture"—it needs proper evaluation.

Too often, patients are reassured with phrases like "give it time" or "it's just inflammation." While patience is required for nerve healing, dismissing these red flags delays critical interventions. Imaging, electrodiagnostics, or referral to neurology may not change the underlying immune process, but they can clarify diagnosis, prevent unnecessary surgeries, and open doors to early rehabilitation. Knowing when to push for more evaluation is part of empowering patients to take control of their care.

Putting Symptoms Into a Map

One way to make sense of the confusing variability is to connect symptoms with their likely nerve roots. Though every case is unique, some patterns recur often enough to guide suspicion:

- **Severe shoulder pain, weakness in abduction, and external rotation** → likely involvement of the suprascapular nerve.
- **Winged scapula with difficulty lifting the arm forward** → long thoracic nerve.
- **Inability to pinch thumb and index finger, difficulty holding small objects** → anterior interosseous nerve.

- **Finger drop without sensory loss** → posterior interosseous nerve.
- **Breathlessness or orthopnea** → phrenic nerve.
- **Hoarseness after acute pain** → recurrent laryngeal nerve.

While this table may look clinical, it is a lifeline for patients and clinicians alike. Knowing that a very specific functional loss correlates to a very specific nerve helps move the conversation away from vague "shoulder injury" toward accurate diagnosis. It also provides a tangible way to track recovery—when a patient can finally form the "OK" sign again or lift their arm without the scapula jutting out, progress is measurable.

The Emotional Overlay

Symptoms are not just physical events. Pain that prevents sleep leads to exhaustion, irritability, and despair. Weakness that strips away independence creates frustration and loss of identity. Visible muscle wasting erodes body image and confidence. For many patients, the emotional toll is as heavy as the neurological one. Depression and anxiety are common companions of PTS, not because patients are weak-willed but because the syndrome destabilizes every aspect of daily life. Recognizing the psychosocial dimension of symptoms is critical for holistic care. The next chapters will address this in more depth, but even in the symptom phase it is worth noting: when you feel overwhelmed, you are not alone, and your distress is not "just in your head." It is an understandable reaction to a brutal condition.

Conclusion: Symptoms as Compass Points

To identify Parsonage-Turner Syndrome is to piece together a puzzle whose pieces are pain, weakness, and variability. The sudden, knife-like pain that often strikes at night. The delayed but dramatic weakness tied to specific nerves. The visible atrophy that follows. The bizarre patchwork of involvement that distinguishes it from other conditions. The red flags that demand urgent evaluation. Together, these form a symptom constellation that, once recognized, becomes unmistakable.

In this chapter we have mapped the features that point toward PTS, translating them into plain language and practical markers. The next step is to move from recognition to confirmation: the diagnostic process. Chapter 3 will take us there, guiding you through the tests, scans, and checklists that separate Parsonage-Turner Syndrome from its many mimics and give patients the clarity they need to plan their path forward.

Chapter 3: The Diagnostic Process

If recognizing symptoms is the art of suspicion, the diagnostic process is the science of confirmation. Parsonage-Turner Syndrome, unlike a broken bone on an X-ray or a torn ligament on an MRI, does not usually present itself with a flashing neon sign. It hides behind overlapping conditions, masquerades as more common shoulder injuries, and teases out confusion even in seasoned clinicians. That is why the road to diagnosis can be as frustrating as the condition itself. Many patients find themselves shuffled from one specialist to another—orthopedist, rheumatologist, chiropractor, pain doctor—before landing in the office of someone who finally names the syndrome. Yet there is a pattern to this journey, and when clinicians understand the right sequence of evaluation, the fog begins to lift.

Step One: A Careful Clinical History

The first and most powerful diagnostic tool is still the story the patient tells. A clinician who listens carefully can often identify PTS without a single test. The sudden onset of severe shoulder or arm pain, especially at night, in someone without obvious trauma, followed by weakness that emerges days to weeks later—that is a signature too distinct to ignore. The problem is that too often, busy practices truncate the history to a few bullet points: "shoulder pain after lifting," "rotator cuff strain," "neck sprain." The subtleties of timing, progression, and quality of pain are lost in translation.

When taken carefully, the history distinguishes PTS from many mimics. Cervical radiculopathy, for example, usually causes pain radiating down the arm in a dermatomal distribution, often with tingling or numbness.

Rotator cuff tears usually present after trauma or overuse and cause pain directly tied to movement. PTS pain, by contrast, is abrupt, severe, often nocturnal, and not necessarily movement-dependent. The delayed weakness is the clincher. Asking the patient, "When did you first notice weakness compared to when the pain started?" is one of the most useful questions in the diagnostic arsenal.

Step Two: The Neurological Examination

The physical examination provides the second major pillar of diagnosis. Here, the clinician looks not just for generic shoulder weakness but for nerve-specific deficits. Winged scapula suggests long thoracic nerve involvement. Loss of thumb–index pinch points to anterior interosseous nerve palsy. Finger drop without sensory changes implicates the posterior interosseous nerve. This selective patchwork weakness, coupled with muscle atrophy, is hard to explain by mechanical shoulder injuries alone.

The exam also evaluates reflexes and sensation. While PTS primarily affects motor nerves, some patients report tingling or altered sensation. Reflexes may remain intact, which can help distinguish PTS from root-level injuries where reflexes are often diminished. The key is to document function carefully, not just "strength 4/5," but specific movements that fail. This specificity makes all the difference when recovery is tracked months later.

Step Three: Excluding the Mimics

Because PTS is relatively unfamiliar to many practitioners, patients often undergo extensive testing to rule out other possibilities before the diagnosis is entertained. This is both a blessing and a curse. On one hand, mimics must be excluded: cervical disc herniation compressing a nerve root, shoulder joint injuries, tumors pressing on nerves, infections like Lyme disease, or autoimmune conditions like brachial plexitis secondary to lupus. On the other hand, the shotgun approach delays clarity and sometimes leads to unnecessary surgeries.

Distinguishing PTS from cervical radiculopathy is a frequent challenge. In radiculopathy, pain and weakness usually occur together, following a root distribution, and are often accompanied by numbness and reflex changes. In PTS, pain precedes weakness by days to weeks, and the distribution is patchy, not confined to a single root. Similarly, while rotator cuff tears can cause profound shoulder weakness, they do not cause muscle atrophy of the forearm or fine motor deficits. Careful correlation of history and exam usually prevents confusion—if the clinician knows to look.

Step Four: Electrodiagnostic Testing (EMG and NCS)

Electromyography (EMG) and nerve conduction studies (NCS) are the workhorses of PTS diagnosis. But timing is everything. If performed too early—within the first week or two—they may appear deceptively normal, because nerve injury takes time to manifest as electrical abnormalities. The optimal window for the first study is usually two to three weeks after onset, when denervation changes begin to appear. Follow-up studies can track reinnervation over time, providing objective evidence of recovery or persistent deficits.

During an EMG, a small needle electrode is inserted into muscles to measure their electrical activity at rest and during contraction. In PTS, affected muscles show spontaneous discharges called fibrillations and positive sharp waves, evidence of denervation. As recovery begins, polyphasic motor unit potentials appear, reflecting reinnervation. NCS complements this by assessing the speed and amplitude of nerve conduction. Together, they map which nerves are affected and how severely.

For patients, the experience can be uncomfortable but invaluable. It transforms vague weakness into a documented pattern, confirming the diagnosis and guiding rehabilitation. Clinicians should explain its importance clearly—EMG is not just "another test," but a window into the nervous system's real-time health.

Step Five: Imaging—When Pictures Speak Louder Than Words

Traditional MRI scans of the shoulder or cervical spine often mislead rather than clarify in PTS. They may show incidental findings like disc bulges or partial rotator cuff tears that have nothing to do with the real problem. This is how many patients end up with unnecessary surgeries. But specialized imaging—magnetic resonance neurography (MRN) or high-resolution ultrasound—has changed the game.

MRN can directly visualize nerves, revealing hourglass constrictions, torsions, or focal swelling. These findings confirm that PTS is not always diffuse inflammation but often involves discrete structural lesions. High-resolution ultrasound, in skilled hands, can show the same constrictions dynamically and at lower cost. These images are not just diagnostic—they are prognostic. If a nerve is kinked and shows no signs of recovery months later, surgery may be considered. If nerves appear inflamed but structurally intact, conservative management may suffice.

Figures of hourglass constrictions often astonish both patients and clinicians: nerves narrowed to a string in one segment, swollen upstream, normal downstream. For patients who have felt gaslit by repeated normal MRIs, these images validate their suffering in a profound way.

Step Six: Questions Patients Should Ask

The diagnostic process can feel like a foreign language, but patients can regain agency by asking targeted questions:

- "When is the right time to get my EMG?"
- "Can you order MR neurography or high-resolution ultrasound to check for constrictions?"
- "Could my symptoms be explained by a disc problem or rotator cuff tear instead?"
- "How will you track recovery over time?"
- "When should I seek referral to a neuromuscular specialist or surgeon?"

Asking these questions forces clarity and helps distinguish clinicians who are familiar with PTS from those who are not. It also prevents passive drift through months of uncertainty.

Step Seven: The Value of a Checklist

Because PTS masquerades as so many other things, a structured diagnostic checklist can be invaluable. Did the pain onset abruptly, at night, without trauma? Did weakness appear days to weeks later, in a patchy distribution? Is there visible atrophy? Has EMG confirmed denervation in multiple nerves? Has imaging ruled out structural compressions? If the answers align, the diagnosis becomes clear. Without such a framework, patients risk endless cycles of inconclusive scans and referrals.

A Schematic in Words: The Hourglass Constriction

Imagine a drinking straw pinched in the middle. Fluid builds up on one side, but barely trickles through the other. That is what an hourglass constriction looks like inside a nerve. The outer sheath narrows sharply, the fascicles kink, and conduction halts. In PTS, these constrictions appear spontaneously, not because of external trauma but because of internal inflammatory changes. Seeing them on MRN or ultrasound is like catching the culprit red-handed. They are not present in every case, but when they are, they offer both explanation and opportunity—surgery may restore flow if natural recovery stalls.

The Patient's Perspective

From the patient's seat, the diagnostic process can feel like a never-ending carousel. One week an orthopedist insists it's a rotator cuff tear. The next, a spine surgeon suspects a slipped disc. A rheumatologist orders blood tests, a physical therapist prescribes exercises, and meanwhile the arm grows weaker. It is no wonder patients describe feeling dismissed, doubted, or misled. Naming the syndrome is therefore more than a technical step; it is an act of validation. A diagnosis transforms the narrative from "we don't know what's wrong" to "this is real, it has a name, and there is a path forward." That psychological pivot is often the first real relief patients experience.

Conclusion: Diagnosis as Compass

The diagnostic process for Parsonage-Turner Syndrome is not about ticking boxes or chasing every possible test. It is about recognizing the story, confirming with focused studies, excluding mimics, and identifying structural lesions when present. History and examination remain the foundation, electrodiagnostics provide confirmation, and modern imaging refines prognosis. Together, they create a roadmap that spares patients the wandering, validates their suffering, and points toward treatment and recovery.

With diagnosis in hand, the next question becomes: what is happening in the broader scientific world to change our understanding of PTS? Chapter 4 turns the spotlight toward recent research—imaging revolutions, genetic discoveries, immune triggers, and clinical trials—that are reshaping what we know and how we treat this condition.

Chapter 4: Recent Research Developments

For decades, Parsonage-Turner Syndrome lived in the shadows of medicine. It was that obscure condition you might encounter once in a lifetime if you were a neurologist and never at all if you were an orthopedic surgeon. Patients were told it was "rare," doctors shrugged when asked about prognosis, and textbooks recycled the same lines year after year. But science has not stood still. In the last twenty years, an explosion of research has redefined what PTS is, how it develops, and how we might treat it. These developments are not just academic—they are reshaping diagnosis, opening treatment options, and changing the conversation from mystery to possibility.

The Imaging Revolution

One of the most striking breakthroughs in PTS research has come not from new drugs but from new ways of seeing. Traditional MRI scans often told clinicians little about the true problem. They could reveal shoulder inflammation or disc bulges, but rarely showed why nerves were failing. That changed with the rise of magnetic resonance neurography (MRN) and high-resolution ultrasound. These tools made the invisible visible.

MRN, a specialized form of MRI, can capture nerves themselves in exquisite detail. What researchers began to see astonished them: hourglass constrictions. Instead of diffuse swelling, many PTS patients showed focal kinks, torsions, or strangulations of their nerves. The nerve, once thought to be uniformly inflamed, was in fact structurally narrowed in discrete spots, like a garden hose pinched in the middle. This discovery forced a rethinking of the entire condition. Perhaps PTS was not purely an inflammatory attack but a combination of immune assault and mechanical constriction.

High-resolution ultrasound, in skilled hands, confirmed this. It showed nerves with alternating swollen and narrowed segments, nerves that twisted in ways normal anatomy never would. Because ultrasound can be performed dynamically—watching nerves in motion—it added a layer of detail MRN could not always match. Studies revealed that these constrictions occur in a majority of EMG-confirmed cases, suggesting they are not rare outliers but central to the syndrome's pathology.

This imaging revolution did more than satisfy scientific curiosity. It provided practical benefits. Patients who once endured months of uncertainty now had visual proof of their condition. Surgeons could identify candidates for neurolysis or nerve transfer with greater precision. Researchers gained a tool to map the natural history of recovery. And most importantly, the idea that PTS was a nebulous, unprovable disorder began to dissolve. Seeing really was believing.

Epidemiology Revisited

Another wave of research has demolished the myth that PTS is vanishingly rare. Older literature repeated incidence figures of two per 100,000 per year, reinforcing the idea that most doctors would never see it. But prospective population studies told a different story. When physicians systematically screened patients presenting with acute shoulder pain, they found that roughly one in a thousand each year developed PTS. That is not a footnote—it is a significant public health concern.

This shift has massive implications. It means that thousands of people annually are going undiagnosed, mislabeled with "rotator cuff tears" or "neck sprains," subjected to unnecessary surgeries or months of ineffective therapy. It also means that research funding and awareness must scale accordingly. The "rare disease" label, while sometimes helpful for advocacy, has in this case harmed recognition. Reframing PTS as underdiagnosed rather than rare is one of the most important recent developments, and it is supported by solid data.

Genetics and the Hereditary Form

For years, physicians knew that PTS sometimes ran in families, but the cause remained obscure. Then came the discovery of mutations in the **SEPT9 gene** as the culprit in hereditary neuralgic amyotrophy (HNA), the familial variant of PTS. SEPT9 encodes a protein involved in cytoskeletal organization, essentially helping nerves maintain their structural integrity. Mutations make nerves more fragile, more prone to injury, and more vulnerable to immune attack.

Patients with hereditary PTS tend to have earlier onset, higher recurrence rates, and more widespread involvement—including not just the brachial plexus but also lumbosacral plexuses, cranial nerves, and even the phrenic nerve. Identifying this genetic link has allowed families to receive counseling, recognize patterns, and prepare for possible recurrence. It has also pushed research forward by providing a biological foothold. Scientists can now study how SEPT9 mutations destabilize nerves and explore interventions that strengthen or protect them.

Genetic understanding also reshapes the narrative for patients. Instead of feeling cursed by randomness, those with hereditary PTS can see their condition as part of a defined biological spectrum. Knowledge, while not a cure, brings clarity.

Immune Triggers: Viral, Post-Vaccine, and Beyond

Another major research focus has been the triggers of PTS episodes. Decades of case reports hinted at links: viral infections, vaccinations, surgeries, childbirth, even intense exercise. Modern research has confirmed these associations while adding nuance. Viral illnesses remain the most common trigger, with upper respiratory infections frequently preceding attacks. Vaccination—particularly influenza and more recently COVID-19 vaccines—has been linked in clusters, though it is important to stress that the risk is extremely small compared to the benefits of vaccination. Surgery and childbirth also appear to act as stressors that unmask the condition.

Immunological studies suggest that in idiopathic PTS, the immune system mounts a misdirected attack on peripheral nerves, perhaps mistaking them for viral proteins in a case of molecular mimicry. Evidence of elevated inflammatory markers, T-cell activation, and complement deposition has been documented in some patients. Though the exact cascade remains unclear, the immune fingerprint is undeniable.

This matters for two reasons. First, it reassures patients that their condition is not "in their head" or random bad luck—it has identifiable biological triggers. Second, it opens the door to targeted immunomodulation. If specific pathways can be identified, therapies might one day prevent or blunt episodes. Current research is inching toward this, but for now, the data remain preliminary.

Trials and Emerging Therapies

The lack of randomized controlled trials (RCTs) has long plagued PTS management. Most of what is known comes from observational studies, case series, or expert consensus. But in recent years, clinical trials have begun to appear, small in scale but important in momentum.

One trial (NCT03441347) explored rehabilitation strategies, focusing on how the central nervous system reorganizes after peripheral nerve injury. The findings highlighted that recovery is not just about peripheral nerve regrowth but also about cortical plasticity—the brain learning to rewire around deficits. This insight has shifted rehabilitation toward not just strengthening exercises but also task-specific training, motor imagery, and techniques that harness neuroplasticity.

Steroids remain controversial. Some observational studies suggest early corticosteroids, given within 30 days of pain onset, reduce pain and improve recovery. Others find no significant long-term difference. The absence of large RCTs means the debate continues. IVIG (intravenous immunoglobulin) has been tested in small cohorts with inconclusive results. What is clear is that the immunological basis of PTS makes it a candidate for immune-modulating therapy, and future trials may yet uncover effective regimens.

Surgical interventions, meanwhile, have been studied with increasing rigor. For patients with documented hourglass constrictions and no recovery after several months, neurolysis or nerve transfer has shown promising outcomes. Success depends heavily on timing and patient selection, but surgical series have reported meaningful functional restoration in carefully chosen cases. The message is not that everyone with PTS needs surgery, but that for a subset, the scalpel offers real hope.

What's Changing Right Now

Taken together, these strands of research paint a picture of a field in transformation. PTS is no longer dismissed as ultra-rare. Imaging has revealed tangible lesions. Genetics has clarified familial risk.

Immunology has traced biological fingerprints. Rehabilitation is being rethought through the lens of neuroplasticity. Surgery has emerged as a serious option, not a desperate experiment. Each of these developments chips away at the old narrative of mystery and futility.

For patients, this means something profound: the future is not static. Twenty years ago, PTS was a diagnosis of exclusion, a shrug, and a pat on the shoulder. Today, it is an active area of research, with scientists, surgeons, and therapists pushing boundaries. Awareness campaigns are growing, patient registries are forming, and clinical trials are multiplying.

The pace of change is not as fast as patients deserve, but it is real. And the knowledge that science is marching forward offers hope in a condition that so often breeds hopelessness.

Conclusion: Science as a Source of Hope

Recent research developments in Parsonage-Turner Syndrome have transformed it from an obscure oddity into a condition with structure, patterns, and pathways of treatment. Imaging has unmasked hourglass constrictions. Epidemiology has reclassified it as under-recognized, not ultra-rare. Genetics has explained hereditary cases. Immunology has traced the fingerprints of immune attack. Clinical trials, though still small, are beginning to shape rehabilitation and treatment.

For patients, these advances matter deeply. They provide validation, options, and a sense of trajectory. They remind us that PTS is not stuck in 1948—it is moving forward with modern science. And they prepare the ground for the next chapter of this guide: treatment options. Because knowing what PTS is and how it behaves is only half the battle. The real question is: what can be done about it? Chapter 5 will answer that, laying out the practical choices—from pain management to physical therapy to surgery—that define the pathway of care.

Chapter 5: Treatment Options Available

By the time a patient finally hears the words *Parsonage-Turner Syndrome* attached to their suffering, the next question comes fast and desperate: "So what do we do about it?" This is where the reality of PTS collides with the expectations of modern medicine. People imagine that once a condition is named, there must be a proven treatment protocol waiting—a pill, a procedure, a step-by-step cure. For PTS, the truth is more complicated. There is no single silver bullet. Instead, treatment is a patchwork of strategies, each addressing one piece of the puzzle: the pain, the inflammation, the weakness, the mechanics, and the long-term adaptation. Some approaches are well studied, others are based on consensus and experience, and still others are experimental. The goal is not to promise full reversal, but to outline realistic options that can reduce suffering, restore function, and help patients reclaim agency in a disorder that often feels like it steals it.

Acute Pain Management

The first hurdle is the pain, and anyone who has experienced the acute phase of PTS knows that "pain" feels like too small a word. It is often described as searing, stabbing, or burning, with a relentlessness that breaks sleep and crushes concentration. Managing this pain is critical—not only to reduce suffering, but also to protect the body from the cascade of exhaustion, depression, and maladaptive movement patterns that uncontrolled pain creates.

For most patients, first-line treatment begins with nonsteroidal anti-inflammatory drugs (NSAIDs) such as ibuprofen or naproxen. These can blunt inflammation and ease discomfort, though in many cases they are not nearly strong enough to tame PTS pain on their own. Adjunct medications often step in, particularly neuropathic pain agents like gabapentin, pregabalin, or duloxetine. These target the nerve-driven nature of the pain rather than just inflammation. Muscle relaxants may also be used, though their effect is usually modest.

Opioids are controversial but sometimes necessary in the acute phase. When pain is so severe that a patient cannot sleep or function, a short course of opioid medication can provide a bridge until the storm begins to calm. The key is careful use—time-limited, monitored, and tapered as soon as possible. Regional nerve blocks, delivered by anesthesiologists or pain specialists, are another option. By injecting anesthetic near the plexus, they can temporarily silence the pain and give the patient a reprieve. These blocks are not curative, but for some patients they are life-changing in the moment.

The central truth about acute pain management in PTS is that it is layered. Few patients find relief from a single pill. Relief comes from combinations, from persistence, and from clinicians who take the pain seriously rather than dismissing it as exaggerated.

Immunomodulation: The Role of Steroids and Beyond

Because PTS is triggered by the immune system, it makes sense to consider treatments that modulate immunity. The most commonly used is corticosteroids, usually prednisone. Observational studies suggest that starting prednisone within 30 days of symptom onset may reduce pain intensity and possibly improve recovery, though results are inconsistent. Some patients swear steroids turned the tide for them; others notice little difference. The lack of randomized controlled trials means uncertainty remains. Still, given the low cost and relative safety of a short steroid course, many clinicians consider it reasonable, especially in the earliest phase.

Other immune-directed therapies remain experimental. Intravenous immunoglobulin (IVIG) has been tried in small series, with inconclusive outcomes. Plasmapheresis has theoretical appeal but limited evidence. Biologics targeting specific inflammatory pathways are being explored in related neuropathies, though not yet in PTS. For now, steroids remain the only practical immune-modulating option, and even they come with caveats. Patients must weigh potential side effects—insomnia, mood swings, elevated blood sugar—against uncertain benefits.

The sobering truth is that while immunology has clarified much about the triggers of PTS, it has not yet delivered a proven therapy. That gap fuels frustration but also underscores the importance of continued research.

Rehabilitation: Protecting, Restoring, and Relearning

If pain management addresses suffering and steroids aim at inflammation, rehabilitation addresses the long war: restoring movement and preventing disability. This is where the patient spends most of their recovery time, and where the outcomes are most visibly shaped.

The first stage is protection. In the acute phase, the priority is maintaining range of motion without overstressing vulnerable joints. When nerves stop feeding muscles, biomechanics fall apart. The scapula may wing, the shoulder may freeze, and abnormal compensation patterns can take root. Early physical therapy focuses on gentle range-of-motion exercises, bracing if necessary, and education on posture. The goal is to prevent secondary injuries—not to strengthen paralyzed muscles that cannot yet respond.

As pain subsides and reinnervation begins, therapy shifts toward activation. Therapists encourage muscles to "wake up," often using targeted cueing and techniques to promote recruitment. Scapular stabilization becomes critical, training surrounding muscles to compensate and protect the shoulder girdle. Strengthening proceeds slowly and carefully, respecting the reality that nerves heal on their own timeline. Over-aggressive strengthening risks fatigue and maladaptive strain.

Later, rehabilitation emphasizes endurance, coordination, and reintegration into functional tasks. It is not enough to restore isolated strength; patients must relearn complex movements like lifting, reaching, and carrying without dysfunctional compensations. Occupational therapy may focus on adaptations for daily life—ergonomic changes at work, modified strategies for cooking, dressing, or driving.

The psychosocial role of therapy cannot be understated. A skilled physical or occupational therapist not only guides movement but also provides encouragement, perspective, and accountability. For patients navigating the long uncertainty of PTS, therapy is often the anchor that keeps them moving forward.

Surgical Options: When the Knife Becomes the Lifeline

Surgery is not for every patient with PTS, but for a subset it offers real hope. The key is identifying those with documented hourglass constrictions who show no signs of recovery after several months. For these patients, neurolysis (surgically releasing the constricted nerve) or nerve transfer (rerouting a healthy donor nerve to restore function) can make the difference between permanent disability and meaningful recovery.

Studies have shown that patients with well-identified constrictions who undergo surgery within the right window can regain significant function. The decision is not simple. Surgery carries risks, recovery is demanding, and outcomes are variable. But for those stuck in paralysis months after onset, it can be transformative.

The rise of MRN and high-resolution ultrasound has made surgical decision-making more precise. Surgeons can now visualize the exact site of constriction before entering the operating room. This reduces guesswork and improves outcomes. Still, surgery is best performed by specialists with experience in peripheral nerve procedures, not general orthopedic surgeons. For patients, the key is to ask whether their surgeon has direct experience with neurolysis or nerve transfers for PTS—not just generic nerve surgery.

Table in Words: What We Know / What We Don't

To keep expectations grounded, it helps to summarize treatment reality in blunt terms.

- **What we know:** Pain management helps, though often requires layers of medication. Early steroids may reduce symptoms, but evidence is limited. Rehabilitation is essential and improves outcomes. Surgery can help in select cases with hourglass constrictions.
- **What we don't know:** Whether steroids truly change long-term prognosis. Whether IVIG or other immune therapies work. Why some patients recover fully while others are left with deficits. How to predict recurrence with certainty.

This table, stripped of false optimism, protects patients from the cycle of raised and dashed hopes. It says: here is what we can do, here is what we cannot, and here is where research must catch up.

The Patient Experience of Treatment

Every option listed above is filtered through the lived reality of patients. Pain medications bring side effects: grogginess, dizziness, nausea. Steroids may help but can leave people sleepless and irritable. Physical therapy is vital but slow, demanding patience when progress feels glacial. Surgery offers hope but requires bravery and trust in a system that may have already let patients down. None of it is easy. Yet most patients find that piecing these options together creates a workable path—not a cure, but a strategy for survival and adaptation.

One patient may swear that prednisone saved them. Another may say therapy was the only thing that kept them sane. A third may look back and thank the surgeon who gave them back the use of their hand. The variability mirrors the syndrome itself. There is no universal formula, only a menu of options that must be tailored to each person.

Conclusion: A Toolkit, Not a Cure

The treatment of Parsonage-Turner Syndrome is not about one cure-all intervention. It is about building a toolkit—pain control, immune modulation, rehabilitation, surgery if needed—that together provide the best chance of recovery. Some tools will matter more for some patients than others. The job of the care team is to assemble the right toolkit, adjust it over time, and support the patient through the long journey.

For patients, understanding this toolkit replaces the myth of the magic cure with the truth of incremental progress. It reframes the battle not as all-or-nothing but as a series of small wins: a night of uninterrupted sleep, a return of thumb-index pinch, the ability to drive again.

With treatment options in hand, the next logical question is: what does it look like in real life? How do actual patients experience this syndrome and its therapies? The next chapter, Chapter 6, answers that question by stepping out of the clinic and into the stories of people who have lived through PTS—their struggles, their recoveries, and the lessons they wish they had known from day one.

Chapter 6: Real-Life Experiences

Medical facts can explain the contours of Parsonage-Turner Syndrome, but numbers and anatomy only go so far. The reality of PTS is lived in kitchens and classrooms, offices and gyms, bedrooms and hospital corridors. It is lived in the sleepless nights of searing pain, in the frustration of trying to tie a shoelace with fingers that no longer obey, in the humiliation of needing help with basic tasks that once felt effortless. Clinical language speaks of "acute pain" and "focal weakness," but patients speak of burning nights, wasted muscles, and a long, uneven road back to something resembling normal. That is why hearing real experiences matters. It translates abstraction into empathy, data into understanding. This chapter gathers composite vignettes based on common trajectories of PTS, stories that highlight the struggles, the coping, and the small victories along the way.

Case One: The Fever and the Forgotten Hand

Jacob was thirty-two, a software engineer and recreational runner, when a flu-like illness knocked him out for a week. He recovered—or thought he had—until one night he woke with what felt like a knife stabbing deep into his shoulder. The pain was so intense that he paced the living room at 3 a.m., clutching his arm and trying not to scream. Over-the-counter medications were useless. His doctor told him it was "probably a muscle strain" and advised ice, rest, and ibuprofen.

Within two weeks, Jacob noticed something stranger than the pain. When he tried to make the "OK" sign with his thumb and index finger, nothing happened. His fingers simply would not touch. He dropped his toothbrush, struggled with his computer mouse, and eventually had to stop running because he could not hold a water bottle. A referral to orthopedics brought an MRI that showed only mild wear and tear. Frustrated, he bounced from one appointment to another until a neurologist ordered an EMG. The results revealed anterior interosseous nerve palsy—classic PTS.

Jacob's recovery was slow. He underwent physical therapy, learning awkward new ways to type and adapting with voice recognition software. Small victories marked his progress: the first time he could again hold a fork, the moment he managed to button his shirt without help, the return of his thumb-index pinch after nearly a year. Today, he still has some weakness, but he has adapted. He tells new patients that the hardest part was not the weakness but the months of doubt before anyone named his condition. "Once I had a diagnosis," he says, "I could finally stop blaming myself for being weak and start focusing on what I could control."

Case Two: The Winged Shoulder and the Stolen Confidence

Maria, a forty-six-year-old teacher, developed sudden pain after a weekend of gardening. It started as an ache but escalated into stabbing jolts that kept her awake at night. She assumed she had overdone it, but when her shoulder blade began protruding oddly from her back, her fear grew. "It looked like a wing," she recalls. Her students noticed and teased her. She tried to laugh it off, but the truth was she could not lift her arm to write on the classroom whiteboard.

The diagnosis took months. Orthopedists suspected rotator cuff tears, and she underwent an MRI that showed minor tendon degeneration—an incidental finding that led to recommendations for surgery. She hesitated, and in the meantime was referred to neurology.

There, a high-resolution ultrasound revealed a constricted long thoracic nerve. She was finally diagnosed with PTS.

Physical therapy became Maria's lifeline. Early on, it was frustrating—her serratus anterior muscle would not engage, no matter how hard she tried. Her therapist explained that the nerve was injured, not the muscle, and that time was needed for recovery. She focused on posture, bracing, and compensatory strategies. Progress was painfully slow. But slowly, over a year, her scapula began to stabilize.

The hardest part for Maria was psychological. "I felt deformed," she says. "I didn't want to wear sleeveless shirts. I hated the way my shoulder looked in photos. I lost confidence in front of my students." Counseling and support groups helped her reclaim confidence, reminding her that winging scapula was not a personal flaw but a medical condition. Today she still notices some winging when tired, but she has regained full independence. She calls her journey "a lesson in patience and humility."

Case Three: The Athlete Who Couldn't Breathe

Darius, a twenty-year-old college soccer player, was at the peak of his athletic career when PTS blindsided him. He woke one morning with searing shoulder pain that spread into his chest. He assumed he had strained something at practice, but soon noticed that he was short of breath, unable to take deep breaths during exertion. His coaches grew concerned when he collapsed in exhaustion after a short run.

Multiple evaluations ruled out asthma, pneumonia, and heart problems. Eventually, a neurologist suspected phrenic nerve involvement and ordered imaging. MR neurography confirmed inflammation of the phrenic nerve along with parts of the brachial plexus. The diagnosis: PTS with diaphragmatic paralysis.

Darius underwent a sleep study that confirmed his diaphragm was barely functioning on one side. He was devastated. Breathing—something he had always taken for granted—was now a conscious effort. He feared his athletic career was over. Rehabilitation included not only traditional physical therapy but also pulmonary exercises, sleep adjustments, and pacing strategies. He adapted by switching from competitive soccer to coaching and strength training, channeling his love of sports into new roles.

Years later, he reflects that PTS "stole my sport but gave me perspective." His diaphragm eventually regained partial function, but he never returned to competitive play. Instead, he became an advocate for awareness, speaking to medical students about the importance of recognizing phrenic involvement. "If just one doctor remembers my story when they meet a patient with unexplained shortness of breath," he says, "it will have been worth it."

Sidebar: What I Wish My Clinician Told Me on Day One

Across patient stories, a common theme emerges: not the pain itself, but the lack of information was the most crushing. Many patients say their first weeks or months would have been less terrifying if their clinicians had simply told them:

- This pain will pass, though it is brutal right now.
- Weakness will follow, and it is not your fault—it is the nerve, not the muscle.
- Recovery takes months to years, not days to weeks.
- Small improvements matter. Celebrate them.
- You are not rare, and you are not alone.

Those five sentences, delivered at the start, could save patients months of confusion and despair.

The Patterns Beneath the Stories

Though the details differ—Jacob's fine motor loss, Maria's scapular winging, Darius's breathlessness—the stories share threads. Sudden, unexplained pain. Weeks later, weakness that made no sense. Delayed or missed diagnoses. A long road of therapy and adaptation. Psychological struggles alongside physical ones. And finally, resilience: finding new ways to work, live, and define identity.

These vignettes are not isolated anecdotes; they reflect the real-world variability of PTS. Some patients recover nearly fully within a year. Others live with permanent deficits. Some find solace in support groups; others fight through largely alone. The variability is frustrating but also liberating—there is no "one right way" to experience PTS, no single trajectory that dictates everyone's future. Each journey is unique, but shared enough to foster community.

Conclusion: The Power of Story

Clinical research is essential, but without patient voices, the full reality of PTS remains invisible. Real-life experiences translate clinical jargon into human terms. They validate the suffering, highlight the challenges of diagnosis, and reveal the emotional terrain that no EMG can capture. Most importantly, they remind patients entering this storm that others have survived it, adapted to it, and even found meaning in it.

In the chapters ahead, we will shift back toward the practical. Chapter 7 explores the impact of PTS on daily life—the strategies, adaptations, and adjustments that allow patients to continue working, driving, and living with dignity. If Chapter 6 was about empathy, Chapter 7 is about action.

Chapter 7: Impact on Daily Life

A diagnosis of Parsonage-Turner Syndrome does not remain neatly contained in a neurologist's notes or inside an EMG report. It spills into every corner of daily existence, disrupting routines, redefining what is "normal," and forcing adaptations in ways that most patients could never have imagined before the syndrome arrived. Living with PTS is not just about pain and weakness—it is about learning to navigate a world designed for two strong arms when one of them no longer works the way it used to. It is about adjusting to fatigue, improvising strategies, and rebuilding confidence after the invisible scaffolding of independence has been shaken. This chapter is not about the clinical science of PTS but about its practical consequences—the things patients and families discover in the trenches of daily life and the strategies that make survival possible.

The Shock of Dependency

One of the first impacts patients describe is the loss of independence. Suddenly, simple tasks like dressing, cooking, or driving become monumental challenges. Shirts with buttons turn into enemies. Carrying groceries feels like scaling a mountain. Even turning a key in a lock can seem impossible when fine motor control is gone. For people who have always prided themselves on self-sufficiency, the shift to asking for help can feel humiliating. Spouses, children, or friends may step in, but the emotional weight of dependency often exceeds the physical weight of the tasks themselves.

The first months after diagnosis are particularly raw. Patients are not yet familiar with adaptive strategies and have not yet built the endurance that comes with recovery. For some, this period brings tears in the grocery aisle, frustration in the kitchen, and despair behind closed doors. Recognizing this as a normal stage, rather than a personal failure, is critical. Every patient who has walked this road has stumbled here.

Workplace Challenges and Adaptations

Work is often the next battlefield. PTS does not discriminate between professions. Teachers, carpenters, musicians, office workers—all face unique challenges when weakness, pain, or fatigue intrude. For a teacher, writing on a whiteboard may become impossible. For a carpenter, holding tools is unsafe. For a musician, fine motor control evaporates. Even office workers, seemingly cushioned by desk jobs, find that typing or using a mouse becomes excruciating.

The Americans with Disabilities Act (ADA) and similar laws in other countries provide for workplace accommodations, but many patients are unaware of their rights. Simple adjustments—ergonomic keyboards, speech-to-text software, lighter tools, modified duties—can mean the difference between continued employment and forced leave. Employers often need education, not just about PTS itself but about the fact that recovery is unpredictable and variable. One month an employee may need major support; six months later they may regain significant independence. Flexibility is essential.

The stigma of invisible disability complicates matters. Colleagues may not understand why someone who "looks fine" cannot complete tasks. Supervisors may question whether the condition is real. Patients find themselves caught between overexertion, risking further injury, and underperformance, risking judgment. Advocacy—backed by medical documentation and sometimes occupational therapy evaluations—becomes crucial.

Driving and Safety

Driving is one of the most emotional markers of independence. For many, the realization that they cannot safely control a steering wheel or shift gears is devastating. Weakness in the shoulder or hand can make sudden maneuvers dangerous. Winged scapula or phrenic nerve involvement may compromise posture and breathing behind the wheel.

Some adapt with modifications: steering wheel knobs for one-handed control, automatic transmissions instead of manuals, or vehicle adaptations recommended by occupational therapists. Others temporarily rely on public transportation, ride-shares, or family support. Losing the ability to drive—even temporarily—feels like losing freedom. But regaining it, whether through recovery or adaptation, is one of the most celebrated milestones patients describe.

Fatigue and Energy Pacing

PTS does not only cause weakness; it causes fatigue that permeates everything. Muscles that once worked effortlessly now strain with basic tasks, burning energy reserves far faster. Patients describe feeling "wiped out" after activities as mundane as folding laundry or cooking dinner. Fatigue also comes from poor sleep during the pain phase, and from the emotional labor of living with chronic illness.

Energy pacing becomes a survival strategy. This means deliberately rationing activity, breaking tasks into smaller chunks, and prioritizing what truly matters. It is learning to accept that "good enough" is often the new standard. Ergonomic adjustments help—using lighter cookware, raising work surfaces, reorganizing closets. But the psychological adjustment—accepting that rest is not laziness but strategy—is the real turning point.

Adaptive Equipment and Bracing

Simple tools can transform daily function. Braces that stabilize the scapula reduce pain and improve posture. Adaptive utensils make eating less frustrating. Velcro shoes or magnetic buttons reduce the challenge of dressing. Ergonomic kitchen gadgets reduce strain. Many patients discover a world of adaptive equipment through occupational therapists, online communities, or trial and error.

For some, bracing is temporary, used during the acute phase to support weak muscles. For others, bracing remains a permanent part of life, particularly for scapular winging or wrist drop. Acceptance varies—some embrace braces as lifesavers, others resent them as visible reminders of disability. Over time, most come to see them as tools, no different than glasses for poor vision.

Care Teams and Coordination

Daily life with PTS is rarely managed by a single clinician. Neurologists diagnose, but physical and occupational therapists guide rehabilitation. Pain specialists manage medications and injections. Psychologists or psychiatrists address depression and anxiety. Pulmonologists may step in for phrenic nerve involvement. Sleep specialists may be required if breathing is affected. Coordinating this team is often left to the patient, who becomes the de facto case manager of their own condition.

Patients who fare best are often those who build networks: a neurologist open to collaboration, a physical therapist willing to adapt routines, a supportive primary care physician who keeps the big picture in mind. Advocacy again becomes essential. Patients must learn to speak up, push for referrals, and demand coordination. It is exhausting—but in PTS, self-advocacy is not optional.

The Psychological Burden

Daily life with PTS is shadowed by an invisible companion: uncertainty. Will this get better? Will it come back? Will I always feel this weak? The lack of definitive answers gnaws at patients. Anxiety about the future compounds depression from the present. Even small setbacks—like a flare of pain or an unexpected stumble—can trigger spirals of fear.

Support groups, whether online or in person, provide crucial validation. Patients often describe the relief of finally hearing someone else put words to their experience. "I thought I was crazy until I heard another patient say the exact same thing," is a common refrain. Mental health resources—therapy, counseling, medication when needed—are not luxuries but lifelines. Recognizing the psychological toll is not indulgence; it is essential care.

Family Dynamics

Families are often the unsung players in the story of PTS. Spouses, children, and parents absorb the ripple effects. They pick up tasks, absorb frustration, and sometimes bear the brunt of emotional outbursts. For some families, the experience deepens bonds, creating solidarity. For others, it strains relationships, exposing fault lines. Patients may feel guilt for being a burden; families may feel helpless watching a loved one suffer. Honest communication, counseling, and practical support are critical to preserving relationships.

Living in a Body That Looks "Normal"

One of the cruelest ironies of PTS is that much of its impact is invisible. Unless there is dramatic scapular winging or obvious muscle wasting, patients may look normal to outsiders. This invisibility breeds misunderstanding. "You look fine" becomes a dagger of dismissal. Employers question absences, friends doubt fatigue, family members underestimate suffering. Patients live in the tension of invisible disability, forced to justify limitations again and again.

For many, this invisibility is harder than the physical weakness itself. It erodes self-confidence and fuels isolation. This is why validation—through diagnosis, through support groups, through simply being believed—matters so profoundly.

Conclusion: Survival Through Adaptation

The impact of PTS on daily life is profound, reshaping everything from brushing teeth to holding jobs. Yet across stories and strategies, one truth emerges: adaptation is survival. Patients who embrace pacing, adaptive equipment, workplace accommodations, psychological support, and family communication find pathways to independence, even if different from what they once knew. Life does not return to the same baseline, but it evolves into a new one—sometimes frustrating, sometimes surprising, but often still full of meaning.

This chapter has mapped the terrain of daily life with PTS. The next chapter turns more deliberately to the psychological and emotional aspects—the trauma of sudden pain, the loss of independence, the uncertainty of prognosis, and the mental health resources that can help. If Chapter 7 is about practical adaptation, Chapter 8 is about emotional survival.

Chapter 8: Psychosocial Aspects

If the physical toll of Parsonage-Turner Syndrome is heavy, the psychological weight can feel even more crushing. Pain fades eventually, weakness may improve slowly, but the emotional shockwave reverberates long after the body begins to heal. People enter PTS as independent adults and suddenly find themselves stripped of control—sleepless from pain, unable to perform daily tasks, uncertain about the future. That loss of control creates fertile ground for anxiety, depression, and even trauma-like responses. Yet these psychosocial aspects are often ignored in clinics focused narrowly on EMGs and MRIs. To understand the full burden of PTS, one must look beyond muscles and nerves to the mind and heart of the patient.

The Trauma of Acute Pain

Pain is not just a symptom in PTS—it is an experience so intense it imprints itself like trauma. Patients often recall the acute pain phase in haunting detail, long after it has passed. Waking in the middle of the night drenched in sweat, clutching the arm, pacing the house because lying down makes the agony worse. Some describe screaming into pillows, others collapsing in tears of exhaustion. The unpredictability of the pain—its sudden jolts, its refusal to respond to medication—creates a sense of helplessness that mirrors traumatic stress.

Even after the pain subsides, memories linger. Some patients develop what resembles post-traumatic stress disorder: fear of recurrence, hypervigilance about minor aches, nightmares of the pain returning. They may avoid physical activity, fearing it will trigger another attack.

This psychological imprint is real and deserves recognition. The trauma of acute pain is not simply forgotten when the nerve begins to recover.

Loss of Role and Independence

One of the most devastating psychosocial impacts of PTS is the sudden loss of role. A parent who can no longer lift a child, a worker who can no longer perform their trade, a musician who cannot play an instrument—these are not minor inconveniences but assaults on identity. People define themselves by what they can do, and PTS can strip that away overnight. The emotional fallout is profound: guilt for letting down family, shame for not performing at work, grief for a self that no longer exists.

Independence, once taken for granted, becomes fragile. Needing help with dressing, eating, or bathing triggers humiliation in adults accustomed to autonomy. Patients describe feeling like burdens, apologizing constantly to spouses or children. This erosion of self-image feeds depression, sometimes more powerfully than the physical symptoms themselves.

The Uncertainty Factor

Uncertainty is the constant companion of PTS. Nobody can say with certainty how much function will return, or when. Nobody can guarantee that the syndrome will not recur. Prognosis is variable, and physicians are often forced to say the dreaded words: "We don't know." For patients, this uncertainty is intolerable. Humans crave timelines, endpoints, guarantees. PTS offers none of these.

This uncertainty generates anxiety that infiltrates daily life. Patients monitor every twitch and tingle, wondering if it signals recovery or relapse. They ask endless questions—"Will I ever be normal again?"—and often receive unsatisfying answers. Some adapt to the uncertainty, learning to live day by day. Others spiral into health anxiety, unable to trust their bodies again.

Depression and Anxiety

It is no surprise that depression and anxiety are common companions of PTS. Pain, loss of function, disrupted sleep, and uncertainty create a perfect storm. Patients describe feeling hopeless, irritable, withdrawn. Some lose interest in hobbies or relationships. Others mask their despair but feel it gnawing inside.

Anxiety manifests in many forms: fear of recurrence, social anxiety about appearing "weak" in front of others, panic when faced with tasks that now feel overwhelming. The invisibility of the condition exacerbates this. When friends or coworkers cannot see the disability, they may dismiss it, leaving the patient isolated and invalidated. That isolation deepens anxiety and depression, creating a vicious cycle.

Mental health screening should be standard in PTS care, but it rarely is. Too often clinicians focus only on physical recovery, leaving emotional wounds untreated. Patients must therefore advocate for themselves, asking for referrals to counseling, therapy, or psychiatric support.

PTSD-Like Features

A subset of patients develop symptoms strikingly similar to PTSD. They relive the acute pain in flashbacks, startle easily at minor aches, avoid activities associated with the initial onset, and struggle with hypervigilance. This is not surprising—severe, unrelenting pain is a form of trauma. Add to that the loss of independence and the uncertainty of recurrence, and the parallels become clear.

For these patients, standard PTSD therapies such as cognitive behavioral therapy (CBT), eye movement desensitization and reprocessing (EMDR), or trauma-informed counseling can help. Naming the experience as trauma validates what patients already know: their suffering was not just physical but psychological.

Resources and Support

Patients navigating the psychosocial impacts of PTS benefit immensely from resources. Educational material helps demystify the syndrome. Advocacy organizations like the National Organization for Rare Disorders (NORD) or Orphanet provide patient guides and connect individuals with research opportunities. Support groups—both online and in person—offer spaces where patients can vent, share strategies, and find solidarity.

The challenge is that not all support groups are created equal. Some are moderated and evidence-based, providing reliable information and encouragement. Others devolve into rumor mills, spreading fear and misinformation. Patients must learn to identify healthy communities—those that balance empathy with accuracy. A good rule of thumb is to seek groups affiliated with reputable medical organizations or moderated by clinicians.

Peer Support: The Power of Shared Experience

Perhaps nothing eases the psychological toll of PTS more than meeting another patient who has walked the same path. Peer support normalizes the experience. Hearing someone else describe waking in the night with stabbing pain, or struggling to button a shirt, or feeling dismissed by doctors, creates instant solidarity. "You too?" is one of the most healing questions a patient can hear.

Peer support also provides practical strategies that textbooks never mention. One patient may share the brand of adaptive utensil that made eating possible again. Another may suggest a breathing exercise that eased phrenic nerve symptoms. These exchanges, trivial to outsiders, can transform daily life for patients.

The Role of Mental Health Professionals

Mental health professionals are often underutilized in PTS care, but their role is essential. Psychologists can help patients reframe loss, manage uncertainty, and build coping strategies. Psychiatrists can prescribe medications for depression or anxiety that interfere with recovery. Social workers can connect patients with resources for work accommodations, disability benefits, or family counseling.

What matters most is integration. Mental health support should not be an afterthought but a core part of the care team. Patients deserve clinicians who recognize that PTS is not just a neuromuscular disorder but a life disorder, affecting mind as much as body.

Conclusion: Healing Beyond Nerves

The psychosocial aspects of Parsonage-Turner Syndrome are not side notes—they are central to the lived experience. Trauma from acute pain, loss of role, uncertainty about prognosis, depression, anxiety, and PTSD-like features all shape the journey. Resources, peer support, and mental health professionals provide lifelines, but only when accessed and acknowledged.

Healing from PTS, therefore, is not only about nerve regeneration. It is about emotional adaptation, psychological resilience, and community connection. Patients who address the psychosocial side alongside the physical often fare better—not because their nerves heal faster, but because their spirits do not wither in isolation.

The next chapter shifts our focus outward again, toward the horizon of PTS care. Chapter 9 explores the future: emerging therapies, technological innovations, and advocacy movements that are shaping what PTS management may look like in the years to come.

Chapter 9: Future of PTS Management

When living with Parsonage-Turner Syndrome, it is easy to feel stuck in the present—trapped between yesterday's pain and today's weakness, with tomorrow a fog of uncertainty. Yet science, technology, and advocacy are slowly reshaping the horizon. What was once a neglected syndrome is now gaining attention in neurology journals, clinical conferences, and patient communities. The future of PTS management is not a single miracle cure but a series of innovations—medical, technological, and social—that together promise a better tomorrow for patients. This chapter looks forward, not with false optimism but with grounded hope, examining what may change in diagnosis, therapy, rehabilitation, and public awareness.

Targeted Immunomodulation

For decades, the dream has been to stop PTS in its tracks—quiet the immune system before it burns through the brachial plexus. Corticosteroids have been the blunt tool of choice, but they are scattershot, suppressing everything from inflammation to bone growth. The future may bring more precision. Researchers are studying the immune fingerprints of PTS, mapping which pathways ignite during an attack. If specific cytokines, T-cell populations, or complement cascades can be identified, therapies might be designed to intervene directly.

Already, drugs used in other autoimmune neuropathies are being studied as potential candidates. Monoclonal antibodies that block inflammatory proteins, complement inhibitors that prevent nerve destruction, and oral agents that modulate T-cell activation are all on the research radar. Though trials are still small or preclinical, the trajectory is promising.

Instead of "try prednisone and wait," the future may offer a menu of targeted treatments chosen based on each patient's immune profile.

Precision Rehabilitation

Rehabilitation is not going away—it will remain the cornerstone of recovery. But the way it is delivered may be transformed. Researchers are learning that recovery after nerve injury is not just about muscle reinnervation but about brain plasticity. The brain reorganizes itself to compensate for lost signals, creating new motor pathways. Harnessing this plasticity is the frontier of rehabilitation.

Future rehab may include virtual reality programs that trick the brain into "seeing" and "feeling" movement even before nerves have fully recovered. Robotics and exoskeletons may provide guided motion that prevents maladaptive compensations while strengthening surrounding muscles. Wearable sensors may track joint angles, scapular motion, and endurance in real time, feeding data back to therapists who adjust exercises remotely. Rehabilitation will become less about trial-and-error and more about precision engineering, customized to each patient's deficits.

Earlier Surgical Triage

The discovery of hourglass constrictions has already changed surgical thinking, but the future may push this further. Instead of waiting six to twelve months to see if recovery happens naturally, patients may undergo early imaging triage. If a nerve is clearly constricted and unlikely to recover spontaneously, surgery may be offered sooner, preventing months of wasted time and irreversible muscle loss.

Surgical techniques are also evolving. Nerve transfers—rerouting a healthy donor nerve to restore lost function—are becoming more refined, with microsurgical advances allowing for targeted, minimally invasive procedures. Bioengineered scaffolds may one day bridge gaps or support regenerating nerves. The once radical idea that surgery could help PTS is now mainstream; the future may make it standard practice for specific subgroups.

Technology at Home: Wearables and Tele-Rehab

The COVID-19 pandemic accelerated the rise of telemedicine, and PTS patients stand to benefit enormously from this shift. Tele-rehab platforms already allow therapists to guide exercises over video, reducing the burden of travel for fatigued or mobility-limited patients. In the future, this may be paired with wearable devices that track range of motion, muscle activity, and even respiratory function in real time. Imagine a patient with phrenic nerve involvement using a home spirometer linked to their neurologist's dashboard, or a wearable patch detecting scapular winging during daily activity and suggesting corrective posture exercises.

These technologies do more than collect data—they empower patients. Instead of waiting months between appointments to learn whether progress is occurring, patients could receive daily feedback, transforming rehabilitation from an isolated struggle into a guided, interactive process.

Artificial Intelligence and Data Integration

Artificial intelligence is becoming a buzzword in every field, but in PTS it has real potential. By analyzing data from EMGs, MRNs, and wearable sensors, AI algorithms may be able to predict recovery trajectories more accurately than any single clinician. They could identify which patients are most likely to benefit from steroids, which are candidates for surgery, and which will recover with conservative care.

Patient registries, powered by AI, may also reveal hidden patterns—subtle triggers, genetic markers, or lifestyle factors that increase risk. For patients who now live in uncertainty, these predictive tools could transform prognosis from guesswork into guidance.

Advocacy and Awareness

Science alone cannot transform PTS care—awareness must rise alongside it. Advocacy movements are already pushing to reclassify PTS not as "rare" but as underdiagnosed. Patient networks are growing, sharing information through social media, podcasts, and online communities. Advocacy organizations are lobbying for insurance coverage of MR neurography and high-resolution ultrasound, pushing for earlier referrals to neurology, and demanding that PTS be included in medical education curricula.

The future may see PTS awareness campaigns similar to those that transformed understanding of fibromyalgia or multiple sclerosis. The goal is not pity but recognition—that when a patient walks into urgent care with sudden shoulder pain, PTS is on the differential, not dismissed as a pulled muscle. Advocacy, though less glamorous than genetic breakthroughs, may ultimately save more patients from months of misdiagnosis.

Insurance and Access

No discussion of the future is complete without confronting the realities of healthcare systems. Right now, many patients are denied access to MR neurography, advanced rehabilitation, or surgery because insurers deem them "experimental" or "unnecessary." The more research validates these interventions, the harder it will be for insurers to refuse coverage. Patient advocacy groups are already collecting data to demonstrate cost-effectiveness: preventing unnecessary rotator cuff surgery, reducing disability claims through earlier rehab, and restoring function through timely surgery.

The future may bring standardized care pathways endorsed by professional societies, making it harder for payers to deny coverage. For patients, this could mean less time fighting on the phone and more time actually healing.

Global Collaboration

PTS research has historically been fragmented—small case series in Europe, isolated trials in Asia, scattered imaging studies in the U.S. The future lies in global collaboration. International registries, pooling data from thousands of patients, will generate statistical power that no single center can achieve. Clinical trials spanning multiple countries can finally test steroids, IVIG, or biologics at scale. Collaborative platforms can share imaging protocols, rehabilitation templates, and surgical outcomes.

For patients, global collaboration means faster answers. Instead of waiting decades for consensus, breakthroughs could emerge within years.

Patient-Reported Outcomes and Empowerment

In the future, research will increasingly value patient-reported outcomes—what patients say matters most. It is not just about EMG scores or muscle strength grades. It is about whether a patient can cook dinner without exhaustion, drive without fear, or sleep without stabbing pain. Tools like the QuickDASH and patient-reported quality-of-life scales will take center stage, guiding both clinical care and research priorities.

Empowered patients will also shape research more directly. Already, patient advocates sit on advisory boards for clinical trials, ensuring that studies reflect real needs. In the future, this partnership will deepen, making PTS care not just doctor-driven but patient-informed.

Conclusion: A Horizon Worth Watching

The future of Parsonage-Turner Syndrome management is not a fantasy of instant cures but a tapestry of incremental progress. Targeted immunomodulators promise to quiet the storm at its source. Precision rehabilitation and technology offer smarter paths to recovery. Earlier surgical triage may save function once thought lost. Wearables and tele-rehab bring care into homes. AI may predict outcomes with clarity. Advocacy and insurance reforms promise access and recognition. Global collaboration and patient empowerment ensure that the syndrome will no longer hide in the margins.

For patients, this future means fewer months of wandering without answers, fewer nights of doubt about whether anyone understands, and more pathways toward recovery and dignity. The horizon is brighter than the past, even if the journey remains long.

With the future mapped, we now return to the present and the practical. Chapter 10 will focus on decision-making in the here and now—helping patients and families ask the right questions, weigh risks and benefits, and chart realistic expectations. Because even as science evolves, every patient must still navigate the choices of today.

Chapter 10: Making Informed Decisions

Knowledge is power, but knowledge without guidance can also overwhelm. By the time a patient with Parsonage-Turner Syndrome has been diagnosed, they have likely already navigated months of pain, confusion, and medical dead-ends. The natural instinct is to ask, "What do I do now?" Unfortunately, there is no one-size-fits-all blueprint. PTS is a condition of variability: the pain intensity, the nerves affected, the timeline of recovery, and the response to treatments all differ from person to person. That variability means decisions are rarely clear-cut. Instead, patients and families must learn to make informed decisions—decisions that weigh risks and benefits, balance hope with realism, and prioritize quality of life over theoretical perfection. This chapter is about equipping patients with the tools to do just that.

The Art of Asking the Right Questions

One of the most empowering strategies for patients is learning which questions to bring into the exam room. Doctors are trained to answer, but they often answer the questions they think you're asking, not the ones that really matter to your life. Preparing targeted questions ensures clarity and prevents misunderstandings. Among the most important are:

- *When is the best time for me to undergo EMG testing, and how often should it be repeated?*
- *Would MR neurography or high-resolution ultrasound help identify hourglass constrictions in my case?*
- *Do you recommend steroids, and if so, why now? What is the evidence for and against?*
- *At what point should we consider surgical referral if recovery is*

not happening?

- *How will you and I track progress—through strength testing, patient-reported outcomes, or both?*
- *What are the red flags that should make me return immediately?*

Asking these questions transforms the visit from a passive experience into an active collaboration. It reminds clinicians that you are not just a set of test results—you are a person who needs clarity, context, and a plan.

Weighing the Risks and Benefits

Every intervention in PTS comes with trade-offs. Steroids may help some patients but can cause insomnia, mood swings, or high blood sugar. Opioids can blunt unbearable pain but carry the risk of dependence. Physical therapy restores function but can feel like endless repetition with slow gains. Surgery can rescue nerves trapped in constrictions, but it requires trust in specialized surgeons and carries no guarantees.

Weighing these options means asking not just "Does it work?" but "Does it work for me, now, in my situation?" A construction worker with finger drop may consider surgery more urgently than an office worker who can adapt with assistive technology. A patient with severe diabetes may decide steroids are not worth the risk of destabilizing blood sugar. A parent caring for children may prioritize pain control above all else to remain functional. The point is not to find the "right" universal answer but the "right-for-you" answer, tailored to your life circumstances.

Understanding the Timeline

Perhaps the most common misstep in PTS decision-making is unrealistic timelines. Patients often expect recovery to happen in weeks. When it doesn't, they feel despair. Clinicians sometimes worsen this by saying "just give it time," without explaining what "time" really means.

Realistic timelines matter. Pain may last weeks. Weakness may emerge after pain fades and persist for months. Nerves regenerate at roughly one millimeter per day, meaning months for noticeable change and often a year or more for meaningful recovery. Even then, residual deficits are common. Knowing this prevents the disappointment of false expectations. Instead of measuring progress week to week, patients learn to measure month to month, celebrating small victories like regaining the ability to hold a cup or lift an arm overhead.

Tracking Outcomes: Beyond Muscle Grades

Doctors often track recovery using the Medical Research Council (MRC) grading scale, which rates muscle strength from 0 to 5. While useful, it reduces complex lived experience into a single number. Patients benefit from adopting broader outcome measures. Tools like the QuickDASH questionnaire capture disability in daily activities. Patient-set goals—"I want to be able to drive again," "I want to cook dinner without exhaustion"—are even more powerful.

Tracking outcomes this way reframes recovery. A patient may still score "3 out of 5" in shoulder abduction but may have regained the ability to put on a coat independently. That functional milestone matters more to quality of life than an abstract number. Keeping a journal of small wins—like fastening a button, sleeping through the night, or writing legibly—reminds patients that progress is happening even if EMG results are slow to change.

The Role of Second Opinions

PTS is often misdiagnosed or under-recognized, so second opinions are not just acceptable—they are wise. Patients should not feel disloyal or guilty for seeking another perspective. In fact, many neurologists encourage it. A second opinion can confirm diagnosis, clarify treatment strategies, or provide access to specialized imaging or surgical expertise not available locally.

The key is to seek second opinions from clinicians with real experience in PTS or peripheral nerve disorders. Not every orthopedist or neurologist will have that expertise. Academic medical centers or neuromuscular clinics are often better bets than general practices.

Balancing Hope with Realism

One of the hardest decisions in PTS management is how much hope to hold. Patients crave certainty—"Will I get better?"—but clinicians cannot provide guarantees. Too much optimism risks crushing disappointment; too much realism risks despair. The balance lies in acknowledging variability while focusing on possibility. Most patients recover some function. Many recover enough to live independently. Residual deficits are common, but adaptation is possible.

Hope does not mean denial. It means focusing on what *can* improve, what *can* be adapted, and what *can* be celebrated along the way. Realism means preparing for the possibility of ongoing challenges while refusing to let them define identity or worth.

Involving Family in Decision-Making

PTS is not suffered in isolation. Families absorb its ripple effects. Decisions about treatment therefore involve not just the patient but their support system. Spouses may help manage medication side effects, drive to therapy sessions, or adjust household responsibilities. Children may adapt to seeing a parent less physically capable. Involving family in decision-making fosters understanding and reduces resentment. When loved ones hear directly from clinicians about prognosis and limitations, they are less likely to doubt or dismiss the patient's experience.

The Psychology of Choice

Decision-making in PTS is not purely rational. Fear, frustration, and exhaustion color every choice. A patient in acute pain may demand surgery immediately, while one in prolonged weakness may reject further interventions out of despair. Recognizing the psychological weight of decisions is part of making them wisely. Mental health professionals can help patients process feelings so choices are made from clarity, not desperation.

Checklists for the Journey

Many patients benefit from written checklists to guide decisions at different stages:

- **Early phase (pain dominant):** Ask about steroids, pain control, and red flags requiring urgent attention.
- **Intermediate phase (weakness/atrophy dominant):** Ask about EMG timing, imaging for constrictions, and rehabilitation strategies.
- **Late phase (recovery/adaptation):** Ask about functional goals, adaptive equipment, surgical referrals if no improvement, and recurrence counseling.

Having these checklists transforms chaotic appointments into structured conversations. They also empower patients to leave with clear next steps rather than vague reassurances.

Conclusion: Decisions as Daily Practice

Making informed decisions in Parsonage-Turner Syndrome is less about one big choice than about a thousand small ones. When to seek imaging. Whether to try steroids. How aggressively to push therapy. When to consider surgery. How to track progress. How to balance hope with realism. Each decision builds upon the last, creating a pathway that is unique to each patient.

The ultimate message is this: patients do not need to make decisions alone, nor should they hand decisions entirely to doctors. Shared decision-making—where patients bring their goals and values, and clinicians bring their expertise—is the strongest foundation. With the right questions, realistic expectations, and functional outcome tracking, PTS management becomes less a maze and more a map.

Having laid the groundwork for decision-making, we now turn outward again. Chapter 11 explores what it means to engage with the broader community: building connections with advocacy groups, contributing to research, and using awareness as a tool of empowerment.

Chapter 11: Engaging with the Community

Parsonage-Turner Syndrome is an isolating condition by nature. It does not have the public recognition of multiple sclerosis or the fundraising machinery of cancer research. Most people have never heard of it, including many doctors. Patients often describe the loneliness of telling coworkers or family about their diagnosis and being met with blank stares. Yet isolation is not inevitable. The last decade has seen a slow but steady growth of patient networks, advocacy organizations, and research initiatives that pull individuals out of solitude and into community. Engaging with this community does more than provide comfort—it empowers patients, advances research, and builds awareness that can change outcomes for future generations.

The Power of Connection

The first step in community engagement is often the simplest: meeting another person with the same condition. Patients who have spent months doubting themselves suddenly hear their own story reflected back. "I thought I was the only one," is a common refrain. That validation is transformative. It shifts the narrative from private struggle to shared experience. It turns isolation into belonging.

Online communities play a central role here. Facebook groups, patient forums, and specialized platforms have become meeting grounds for people across the world. Some groups count hundreds of members; others, thousands. In these spaces, patients trade stories, share practical tips, and provide emotional support. One person may post about how they manage scapular winging with a specific brace; another may share the name of a neurologist experienced in PTS; another may simply vent about a rough day. The responses are often immediate and empathetic—people who truly understand because they have lived it themselves.

But connection does not have to be digital. Local support groups, though rarer, provide face-to-face solidarity. Advocacy organizations are increasingly offering regional meetups, webinars, and conferences. These events are more than informational—they are lifelines. Patients leave not only with new knowledge but with friendships that endure.

Credible Sources of Information

In an era of endless online information, not all resources are created equal. Patients engaging with the PTS community must learn to discern credible sources from misinformation. Among the most reliable are:

- **NORD (National Organization for Rare Disorders):** Provides accessible summaries of PTS, patient handbooks, and connections to research initiatives.
- **Orphanet:** An international database of rare conditions, offering detailed medical information.
- **Academic medical centers:** Many publish patient-facing guides or host informational webinars on brachial plexus disorders.
- **Peer-reviewed journals:** For those who want to dive into the science, PubMed provides open access to many PTS studies.

Community forums are invaluable for support, but they are not substitutes for medical advice. Engaging with both peer support and credible scientific sources creates the strongest foundation.

Contributing to Research

One of the most meaningful ways patients can engage is by participating in research. Clinical trials for PTS remain small, but their success depends on patient involvement. Registries that collect patient histories, outcomes, and genetic data are essential to building statistical power. Without patient participation, research cannot progress.

Some patients worry that their contribution is too small to matter. In truth, every data point is valuable. A single EMG report, a single genetic test, a single functional outcome survey adds to the mosaic. Engaging in research also provides patients with early access to innovations—experimental rehabilitation protocols, new imaging modalities, or immune-modulating treatments.

Advocacy organizations and academic centers are increasingly calling for patient-reported outcomes. This means patients do not need to travel to a lab—they can complete surveys online, tracking their recovery and sharing insights. These patient voices are reshaping the field, ensuring that future treatments address not just nerve function but quality of life.

Raising Awareness

Another key aspect of community engagement is advocacy. Awareness is the currency of change. The more people know about PTS, the more likely it is to be diagnosed early, treated seriously, and researched adequately. Raising awareness can happen at many levels:

- **Personal level:** Explaining the condition to friends, family, and coworkers.
- **Professional level:** Sharing educational materials with local doctors, therapists, or support staff.
- **Public level:** Writing blogs, speaking at events, or using social media to amplify patient voices.

Awareness campaigns may seem small—an article in a local newspaper, a patient story shared on a podcast—but they ripple outward. One doctor reading that article may think twice the next time they see a patient with unexplained shoulder pain. One physical therapist hearing that podcast may recognize scapular winging as nerve-related, not just posture-related. Advocacy turns private suffering into public education, multiplying its impact.

Advocacy for Insurance and Access

Engagement also means confronting systemic barriers. Many patients find themselves denied MR neurography, high-resolution ultrasound, or specialized rehabilitation because insurers deem them "experimental." Advocacy organizations are collecting patient stories and economic data to challenge these denials. Patients themselves can contribute by writing appeals, documenting unnecessary costs (such as surgeries later found unnecessary), and joining collective efforts to push insurers for recognition.

At a larger scale, professional societies are beginning to draft standardized guidelines for PTS management. Once published, these guidelines will strengthen patient appeals by providing insurers with authoritative roadmaps. Patient engagement in advocacy ensures that these guidelines reflect lived reality, not just academic theory.

Healthy vs. Unhealthy Communities

While community engagement is powerful, not every group or forum is equally healthy. Some online spaces devolve into fear, negativity, or misinformation. Patients may encounter exaggerated claims, miracle cures, or fatalistic despair. Engaging wisely means evaluating communities by their tone and moderation. Healthy communities encourage evidence-based information, support members' diverse experiences, and celebrate progress. Unhealthy ones spread myths, discourage professional care, and amplify hopelessness.

A practical tip: if a group spends more time promoting unproven supplements than discussing rehabilitation, it is probably not the right space. If members discourage medical consultation, that is a red flag. Healthy engagement means finding communities that lift you up, not drag you deeper into despair.

Templates and Tools for Engagement

Engaging with the community also includes practical advocacy tools. Patients can prepare templates for awareness letters to employers, schools, or local media. These explain PTS in plain language, outline accommodations needed, and provide credible sources. Some advocacy organizations already supply such templates, saving patients the exhausting task of reinventing the wheel.

For example, a workplace letter might explain: "Parsonage-Turner Syndrome is a neurological condition that causes sudden nerve pain, weakness, and muscle wasting. Recovery can take months to years. Accommodations such as ergonomic equipment, flexible scheduling, or modified duties may be needed temporarily or permanently." Tools like this turn private suffering into structured requests for understanding.

The Emotional Benefits of Engagement

Engaging with the community is not only about advocacy and research—it is also a balm for the soul. Patients describe feeling lighter when they share their stories, comforted when they hear echoes of their own struggles, and energized when they help newcomers. Helping others often becomes part of healing. Teaching a newly diagnosed patient what to expect, or sharing which brace worked best, transforms isolation into purpose.

This sense of belonging is powerful. It reframes PTS from a personal curse into a shared journey. It reminds patients that while they may feel rare, they are not alone. In a world where many conditions drown in stigma, community engagement provides both strength and dignity.

Conclusion: From Patient to Advocate

Engaging with the community is the final outward-facing step in the PTS journey. It begins with connection—meeting others who understand. It grows into research participation, advocacy, and awareness campaigns. It evolves into purpose, as patients shift from sufferers to advocates. This is not to say everyone must become a public activist. Engagement can be as simple as posting in a support group, completing a survey, or explaining PTS to one more person who had never heard of it before.

The key message is that engagement matters. It changes lives—your own and others'. It builds the foundation for future treatments, accelerates recognition, and softens the loneliness that comes with invisibility. Patients who engage discover that while their nerves may have betrayed them, their voices still carry power.

With this, we step into the final chapter of the main text. Chapter 12 is about looking forward personally—your journey ahead. It takes the lessons of science, daily life, and community and turns them inward, helping patients set goals, manage recurrence risk, and celebrate progress. Where the previous chapters have looked outward, Chapter 12 brings the focus home.

Chapter 12: Your Journey Ahead

By the time a patient reaches this point—diagnosed, treated, adapting, and hopefully connected to a community—the question shifts from *what now?* to *what next?* Parsonage-Turner Syndrome is not an acute event that ends with a neat bow. It is a journey, often long, sometimes recurring, always life-altering. Chapter 12 is about turning the knowledge of this guide into personal practice: setting realistic goals, preparing for possible recurrence, focusing on long-term adaptation, and recognizing small wins as true victories. Where earlier chapters have mapped science, treatment, and community, this one brings the focus inward—onto the individual patient charting their own road ahead.

Goal-Setting as Compass

In the fog of PTS, goals are not luxuries; they are compasses. Without them, days blur together into cycles of fatigue and frustration. With them, patients regain a sense of direction. Effective goal-setting means breaking recovery into digestible timeframes.

30-day goals often focus on acute management: stabilizing pain, establishing a rehab routine, arranging workplace or family accommodations, and learning the basics of energy pacing. Success in this stage may look like sleeping through the night without breakthrough agony, attending therapy consistently, or mastering one adaptive strategy that reduces daily strain.

60-day goals build on stabilization. By this point, patients may shift toward function: regaining partial range of motion, performing basic tasks independently, or reducing medication reliance. Celebrating small returns—like being able to lift a glass of water with the affected hand—anchors hope in tangible progress.

90-day goals focus on adaptation and integration. Whether or not strength has significantly returned, the patient aims to re-enter roles that matter—returning to work with accommodations, resuming modified hobbies, reconnecting socially. At this stage, "success" does not mean full recovery; it means life is being lived again.

Goals serve another purpose: they make recovery measurable in ways that matter to the patient. A muscle grade of "3 out of 5" may look disappointing on paper, but being able to cook a meal independently feels like triumph.

Preparing for Recurrence

PTS is not always a one-time visitor. Idiopathic cases recur in about one out of four patients. In hereditary PTS, recurrence is even more common, with episodes accumulating over a lifetime. This reality can cast a shadow over recovery. Patients often describe living with a "sword over the shoulder," waiting for the next strike.

Preparation, however, transforms fear into readiness. Patients can build recurrence plans with their care team:

- Knowing early warning signs of relapse and when to seek urgent evaluation.
- Keeping an updated folder of past EMG, imaging, and therapy records for quick reference.
- Identifying a neurologist or clinic familiar with PTS for rapid access.
- Creating a flexible support plan with family or workplace, so sudden disability does not trigger chaos.

Recurrence counseling should also emphasize resilience. Many patients who relapse report that the second time, while still devastating, was less terrifying because they knew what it was and how to navigate it. Knowledge is armor.

The Role of Long-Term Adaptation

Even when recovery is significant, residual deficits are common. Endurance may remain limited, fatigue may strike quickly, fine motor control may never fully return. Long-term adaptation means accepting these truths without surrendering to them. It means embracing adaptive strategies not as temporary crutches but as permanent allies.

Adaptive tools, pacing strategies, ergonomic modifications, and psychological resilience form the pillars of this adaptation. Patients who thrive are those who redefine "normal." Instead of chasing a past self with frustration, they craft a present self that is capable, independent, and purposeful—even if different than before.

Functional Wins vs. Strength Grades

Recovery in PTS often tempts patients into focusing obsessively on strength grades. Every EMG, every manual muscle test becomes a referendum on progress. But nerves do not heal linearly, and muscle grades often lag behind lived experience. That is why focusing on *functional wins* is more powerful.

The first time a patient carries groceries without pain, or lifts a child again, or types without fatigue—these are milestones more meaningful than numbers. Keeping a "victory journal," noting these wins, reframes recovery from despair into momentum. Over time, the journal becomes a record of resilience.

The Emotional Arc of Moving Forward

The journey ahead is not purely physical. Emotionally, patients often travel through phases: grief at the onset, anger during pain, despair during weakness, cautious hope during recovery, and finally, acceptance and adaptation. This arc is not linear—patients may cycle through stages repeatedly, especially if setbacks occur. Recognizing the arc as normal prevents self-judgment.

Mental health support remains vital long after acute phases pass. Counseling, peer support, and mindfulness practices help patients integrate the experience into identity without letting it dominate. Moving forward emotionally means recognizing both the scars and the strength gained.

Building Resilience into Lifestyle

PTS recovery is not about returning to the exact same life as before but about building resilience into the one that follows. Patients often find that lifestyle changes improve not only their recovery but their overall well-being:

- Prioritizing sleep hygiene, since fatigue worsens symptoms.
- Maintaining gentle but regular physical activity to prevent deconditioning.
- Managing stress, which may exacerbate pain and fatigue.
- Balancing work and rest to preserve energy for what matters most.

In this way, the journey ahead is not only about surviving PTS but about reshaping life in ways that promote health and resilience across the board.

Recurrence Does Not Mean Defeat

For those who face recurrence, it is important to remember that relapse is not failure. It does not erase past progress or negate resilience. Each episode is unique; some are milder than the first, some affect different nerves, some resolve more quickly. Having a recurrence plan, support networks, and established adaptive strategies makes subsequent episodes more manageable. Patients who frame recurrence as "another chapter" rather than "the end of the story" retain agency even in the face of relapse.

Celebrating Small Wins

PTS recovery is rarely dramatic. It does not unfold like a sudden miracle. It creeps in increments—a flicker of muscle activation, an extra hour of stamina, a smoother reach overhead. Patients who learn to celebrate these small wins find greater resilience. This is not toxic positivity—it is survival strategy. Recognizing progress, however small, builds momentum against despair.

One patient described the joy of being able to tie his shoes again after nine months. Another celebrated typing a full page without fatigue. These moments, insignificant to outsiders, are monumental for those living with PTS. Building rituals of celebration—sharing wins in support groups, journaling them, or marking them with personal rewards—keeps the journey bearable.

Conclusion: Walking Forward with Courage

The journey ahead with Parsonage-Turner Syndrome is neither simple nor predictable. It demands patience, adaptation, resilience, and community. It asks patients to set realistic goals, prepare for recurrence without being paralyzed by it, redefine success in terms of function rather than perfection, and celebrate progress as it comes. It is not a straight road but a winding one, yet many have walked it before, and many will walk it after.

Your journey ahead is not about returning to who you were before PTS. It is about becoming who you are after it—someone who has endured pain, adapted to loss, and learned resilience. This is not to romanticize suffering but to recognize survival. The syndrome may scar nerves, but it does not have to scar identity.

With this, the core chapters of this guide draw to a close. The appendices that follow provide practical tools: differential diagnosis tables, rehabilitation templates, imaging request phrasing, surgical questions, and accommodation letters. These are the nuts and bolts—the quick references to support the long road you are walking. But the most important resource remains your own resilience, shaped by knowledge, bolstered by community, and carried forward step by step.

Appendices

Appendix A: Differential Diagnosis Table

One of the greatest challenges with Parsonage-Turner Syndrome is that its early symptoms overlap with many other conditions. Shoulder pain and weakness are not uncommon complaints in medical practice, and unless clinicians know how to differentiate PTS, patients may be misdirected into months of ineffective or unnecessary treatments. This appendix outlines the most common conditions confused with PTS, highlighting the distinguishing features that separate them.

- **Cervical Radiculopathy:** Pain radiates along a dermatomal distribution, often accompanied by numbness or tingling in the hand. Weakness appears simultaneously with pain, rather than weeks later. Reflexes are often diminished.
- **Rotator Cuff Tear:** Pain is linked to movement and injury history, weakness is mechanical rather than nerve-driven, and muscle wasting is localized to the shoulder. Imaging usually confirms.
- **Adhesive Capsulitis (Frozen Shoulder):** Severe stiffness dominates rather than focal weakness. Pain limits range of motion globally, not in specific muscle groups.
- **Brachial Plexus Tumor or Mass Lesion:** Progressive rather than abrupt onset. Often associated with systemic signs such as weight loss. MRI reveals compressive mass.
- **Infection (Lyme, Herpes Zoster):** May mimic PTS pain, but serologies or skin lesions (in shingles) give clues.
- **Stroke or Central Lesions:** Weakness is sudden but associated with other neurologic deficits—speech, vision, gait—unlike isolated PTS.

For patients, this table is a reminder that misdiagnosis is not their fault. For clinicians, it underscores why careful history and timing of weakness are essential.

Appendix B: Rehabilitation Progression Templates

Rehabilitation for PTS is not a one-size-fits-all endeavor. It evolves with time, from acute pain to reinnervation. This appendix provides a structured progression, not as a rigid recipe but as a guide that patients and therapists can adapt.

Acute Phase (0–6 weeks):

- Focus on gentle range of motion to prevent joint stiffness.
- Use supportive bracing if scapular winging threatens shoulder mechanics.
- Pain control prioritized—avoid strengthening paralyzed muscles.

Subacute Phase (6–24 weeks):

- Begin targeted activation of reinnervating muscles.
- Emphasize scapular stabilization and posture correction.
- Use tactile or visual cues to encourage recruitment of weak muscles.
- Prevent maladaptive compensations (e.g., shrugging shoulder instead of true abduction).

Reinnervation Phase (6–18 months):

- Introduce strengthening, starting with low resistance, high repetition.

- Build endurance gradually—fatigue is a real barrier.
- Functional retraining: practice lifting, reaching, fine motor tasks.

Adaptation Phase (long-term):

- Integrate adaptive tools for persistent deficits.
- Focus on energy pacing, ergonomics, and lifestyle modification.
- Continue monitoring for recurrence or contralateral involvement.

Therapists often stress patience: nerves heal on their own timeline. Pushing too hard too soon can do more harm than good.

Appendix C: Imaging Request Phrasing

Patients often struggle to get appropriate imaging. Insurance denials and clinician unfamiliarity create barriers. This appendix provides language that patients or doctors can use when requesting advanced imaging.

- **For MR Neurography:**
  "Evaluate for focal nerve constrictions or hourglass lesions in the brachial plexus and peripheral nerves. Patient with clinical suspicion of Parsonage-Turner Syndrome. Prior EMG confirms multifocal denervation."
- **For High-Resolution Ultrasound:**
  "Request high-frequency probe imaging of affected brachial plexus branches to assess for focal constrictions, torsion, or nerve swelling. Correlate with EMG findings."

Precise language helps radiologists know what to look for and insurers understand medical necessity. Patients can carry these templates into appointments as advocacy tools.

Appendix D: Surgeon Questions for Constriction Lesions

For patients referred to surgery after PTS, clarity is everything. This appendix lists questions patients should ask before agreeing to procedures:

1. How many PTS or brachial plexus constriction cases have you operated on?
2. Do you perform neurolysis, nerve transfer, or both?
3. How do you decide when surgery is appropriate?
4. What outcomes can I realistically expect—and what percentage of your patients achieve them?
5. What are the risks of worsening function or persistent pain?
6. How soon after surgery can rehabilitation begin?
7. If this surgery does not restore function, what are the next steps?

These questions separate experienced peripheral nerve surgeons from generalists. Patients should not hesitate to walk away from surgeons who cannot answer confidently.

Appendix E: Work and School Accommodation Letters

Daily life with PTS often collides with rigid expectations at work or school. This appendix provides sample language for requesting accommodations.

Workplace Template:

"To Whom It May Concern:

[Patient Name] has been diagnosed with Parsonage-Turner Syndrome, a neurological condition causing sudden severe pain, muscle weakness, and fatigue. Recovery can take months to years, and functional limitations vary. Temporary or permanent accommodations may include: modified duties, flexible scheduling, ergonomic equipment, or assistive technology. These accommodations will enable [Patient Name] to continue contributing effectively while managing medical needs."

School Template:

"To School Administration:

[Student Name] is under medical care for Parsonage-Turner Syndrome, which affects nerve function and muscle control. This may limit writing, carrying, or participating in physical activities. Accommodations may include extended time for assignments, access to note-taking support, reduced physical load, and flexible participation in physical education. These adjustments ensure equal educational opportunity while the student recovers."

Letters like these provide structure for conversations that might otherwise feel awkward or adversarial. They frame PTS as legitimate and deserving of accommodation, reducing stigma.

Conclusion: Tools for the Road Ahead

The appendices are not narrative—they are maps, templates, and scripts. They exist to save patients from reinventing the wheel, to arm them with language that insurers and institutions respect, and to guide clinicians unfamiliar with the syndrome. Where the earlier chapters told the story of PTS—the history, the symptoms, the treatments, the future—these appendices provide the nuts and bolts of living with it.

Parsonage-Turner Syndrome will continue to test patience, resilience, and adaptation. But with the right tools, patients can navigate more confidently. Whether it is handing an imaging request to a radiologist, showing a checklist to a therapist, or sending an accommodation letter to a school principal, these practical aids turn knowledge into action.

With this, the guidebook closes—not with false promises of cures, but with hard-earned clarity, compassion, and resources. The journey remains long, but it is no longer traveled alone, and it is no longer without a map.

www.ingramcontent.com/pod-product-compliance
Lightning Source LLC
LaVergne TN
LVHW022308200926
848481LV00004B/1244
* 9 7 9 8 2 3 0 1 1 7 1 6 2 *